THE STRANGE CASE OF
DR. COUNEY

blue
rider
press

ALSO BY DAWN RAFFEL

In the Year of Long Division

Carrying the Body

Further Adventures in the Restless Universe

The Secret Life of Objects

THE STRANGE CASE OF
DR. COUNEY

*How a Mysterious European Showman
Saved Thousands of American Babies*

DAWN RAFFEL

BLUE RIDER PRESS

New York

blue
rider
press

An imprint of Penguin Random House LLC
375 Hudson Street
New York, New York 10014

Copyright © 2018 Dawn Raffel
Penguin supports copyright. Copyright fuels creativity, encourages
diverse voices, promotes free speech, and creates a vibrant culture.
Thank you for buying an authorized edition of this book
and for complying with copyright laws by not reproducing, scanning,
or distributing any part of it in any form without permission.
You are supporting writers and allowing Penguin to
continue to publish books for every reader.

Blue Rider Press is a registered trademark and its colophon
is a trademark of Penguin Random House LLC

Pages 283–284 constitute an extension of this copyright page.

ISBN 9780399175749

Printed in the United States of America
1   3   5   7   9   10   8   6   4   2

Book design by Amy Hill

For the babies

CONTENTS

Part Three
THE BLACK STORK

THE STRANGE CASE OF
DR. COUNEY

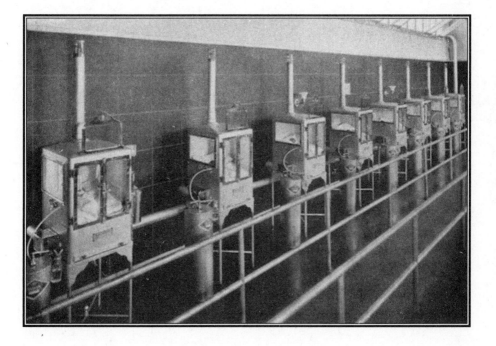

PROLOGUE: BREATH

The pains came too early. The cramping of the womb. The ragged breaths. The life demanding release. The woman, Marion Conlin, was carrying twins, and on an otherwise gentle Thursday in May, her labor had commenced. Too soon. Not now. Not yet. Each contraction a blow.

Only the year before, she and her husband, Woolsey, had celebrated their wedding. Summer of 1919. Atlantic City honeymoon, where, in that golden pocket—the Great War over, Prohibition not begun—a newlywed couple might sip champagne and hear their beautiful fortunes told and stroll in their swim suits into the sea, laughing.

Now they were in a hospital in Brooklyn. Marion's labor could not be stopped. One daughter entered the world, drew breath for twenty minutes, and lay still. The second was so tiny, it was painful to look, her skin near translucent.

The obstetrician had no words of comfort. He gestured toward the child who had died. "Don't rush to bury that one," he said bluntly, "because you will need to bury the other one too."

"But she's alive," Woolsey said.

"She is not going to live the day."

This was too much to bear. "Well, she's alive *now*," her father said. In

THE STRANGE CASE OF DR. COUNEY

Atlantic City, he had seen a sideshow on the boardwalk with premature infants in incubators, being saved. "Aren't there machines for little babies that will help them?"

"Yes, but we don't have those here," the doctor said. "And anyway, it wouldn't make a difference in this case because she is not going to live."

Atlantic City was hours, lifetimes, away, but something Woolsey Conlin had heard came back to him: That boardwalk doctor ran another sideshow, closer to home. While the obstetrician continued to insist on the hopelessness of the situation, Woolsey Conlin picked up his two-pound daughter, wrapped her in a towel, walked outside, and hailed a taxi. "Coney Island," he told the driver. "Can you step on it, please?"

Part One

MASTERS OF INVENTION

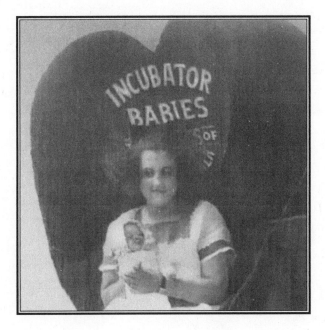

"ALL THE WORLD LOVES A BABY"

Chicago, 1934

Chicago had already sweated through one hell of a week, and today was only Wednesday. The trouble began with a bang, literally, on Sunday when the cops shot down John Dillinger outside the Biograph. Gangster was seeing a movie. If you didn't know better, you might have believed the deceased was seeking revenge: As the final larcenous breath rattled out of his lungs, the city was being strangled.

By Tuesday, the mercury in the snazzy Havoline Thermometer Tower, soaring over the Century of Progress fairgrounds on the lakefront, had shot up to 105—with 109 degrees reported inland at the airport. Either way, it was the hottest day ever on record for Chicago.

Heat deformed the air, which seemed to wobble. Clothes stuck to flesh. Flesh stank. With ice in short supply and the stench of the slaughterhouses ripening—where pigs strode doomed over the bridge of sighs and cattle hung bloody from hooks—people fled to the beaches of Lake Michigan to sleep.

During the day, perspiring throngs pressed their way into the Great Halls and pavilions at the world's fair, less interested in the scientific and cultural marvels on display than in inhaling refrigerated air. They poured out onto the midway, dripping into their summer cottons and brimmed hats, fanning their faces with folded maps, mopping up ice cream that melted faster than they could eat. Freaks, savages, steamy strippers, and miniature humans were there for their viewing pleasure. If people couldn't stanch the sweat, they could at least secure a couple of hours' respite from the cruel Depression and the news coming out of Germany.

Today, the high—finally!—was supposed to be south of 100. That in itself was cause for celebration. As for the news, for the fifteen minutes between 12:45 and 1:00 p.m., the airwaves would belong to Dr. Martin Arthur Couney and the adorable babies whose lives he had saved in his incubator sideshow.

The radio script had a written instruction not to conduct today's program as a farce. Yes, the announcer could make a few cracks about all the crying and yelping, but he needed to mind himself, on account of the "ethical standing" of the city's physicians who had a manicured hand in this thing. This baby "homecoming" would not be half as fun as the midget wedding two weeks earlier. Why, even a former vice president of the United States had been out in the Lilliputian village when that tiny torch singer married her groom, and the cops had to stop the mob from going nuts.

Every day, you had a new extravaganza at the Century of Progress. It wasn't just the grand Hall of Science, the Halls of Religion, and Travel and Transport, the Homes of Tomorrow, with everything prefabricated, some kind of dream. It was Ripley's and strippers and marching bands and neon Deco blazing through the sweltering night. So what if it wasn't as grand as the famous White City back in 1893? Who cared if the old folks didn't find the sky ride quite as stirring as the Ferris wheel they liked to carry on about? You really had to hand it to the planners and the backers—they'd managed to pull a rabbit out of the hat of the Depression.

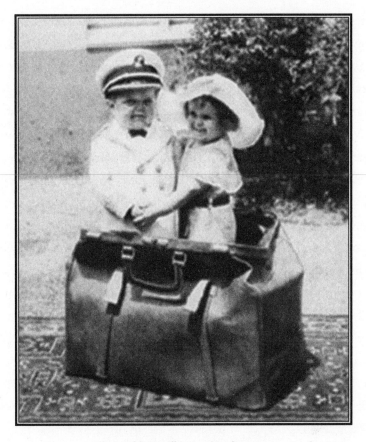

The world's smallest man and women,
at the Century of Progress.

Given a choice, you might rather escape than eat. People jam-packed the midway, reeking of Tabu perfume, of Burma-Shave, and summer BO, ready to part with whatever they had, dollars thick in silver clips or crumpled in a pocket, a scavenged coin or two, nickels pilfered from a pay phone.

Train after train steamed into Union Station, belching out tourists. Folks at home depended on the radio, the ticket to the world. Today's show would reconvene the tots who'd been the littlest humans breathing, premature babies so small you could scarcely imagine a heart, a lung, a soul. They'd spent the summer of '33 sleeping and cooing in Martin

Couney's sideshow on the midway. "Infant Incubators with Living Babies"—the sign so big you'd have to be dead to miss it. Just next door, inside the Streets of Paris, Sally Rand was doing her scandalous fan dance that made her look naked, but Martin Couney had something most of these people had never seen before.

Saving a two-pound person was a neater trick than swallowing a dagger or eating a flame. Most hospitals were not equipped to do it. And even if they were, you couldn't barge in off the street. So every day, the crowds paid a quarter to see the preemie sideshow. Housewives, dressed up in their prettiest slim-waist prints, salesmen who'd blown into town from Topeka and Canton and Scranton on a junket, school-marms in their sensible shoes, the farmhands and the factory men, swoony schoolgirls dragging the boys from the block, society gals in their slouchy hats, stenographers and operators, grannies and aunties and sticky brats. With luck, they got to watch the nurses feed or bathe the

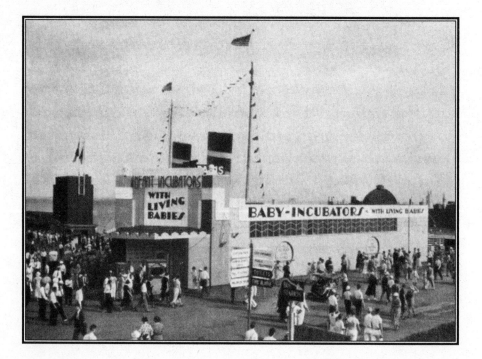

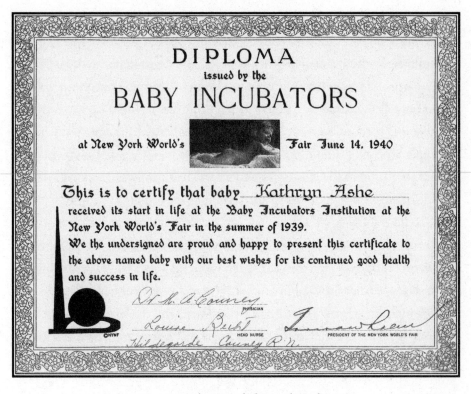

DIPLOMA

issued by the

BABY INCUBATORS

at New York World's   Fair June 14, 1940

This is to certify that baby _Kathryn Ashe_
received its start in life at the Baby Incubators Institution at the
New York World's Fair in the summer of 1939.
We the undersigned are proud and happy to present this certificate to
the above named baby with our best wishes for its continued good health
and success in life.

PHYSICIAN

HEAD NURSE   PRESIDENT OF THE NEW YORK WORLD'S FAIR

Martin continued issuing diplomas through 1940.

patients. The French nurse, Madame Recht, would flash a diamond ring and slip it over an infant's wrist, all the way up its skinny arm, to demonstrate scale.

Today, the "graduates" included forty-two "lusty-lunged boys and girls of all nationalities and assorted colors," according to the press release. Singles, twins, a sole surviving triplet. Plus, a VIP: Miss May Winter, class of '01, from Dr. Couney's show at the Buffalo World's Fair. Thirty-three-year-old spinster worked in the travel department at Carson Pirie Scott & Co.—point being, she was normal. Productive. These babies could grow up to be like anybody else. They didn't have to die.

Martin Couney had been selling this idea forever. Anyone who'd ever bought a pickle in Atlantic City or spent a salty day at Coney Island had heard of this guy. Babies came straight from the bloody birthing beds and overburdened hospitals—infants who doctors swore would die, or swore would die without him. No other hope. Back in the aughts, before half of these people remembered, he used to exhibit in Chicago's fun-parks. Jolly kind of fellow. European. Pretty much everyone thought he was swell. Excepting some of the members of the medical establishment. Many had simply ignored him. Others were made uneasy—the way he practiced next to the din of the chute-the-chutes and freak shows, making a spectacle of the weaklings, even if he saved them.

Today's show could change his reputation. At a quarter of one—live from the Century of Progress!—two unimpeachable doctors would join him on the midway and publicly agree about the way to save these babies. No, not with sideshows, but yes, with incubators—as Martin had been saying all along—and yes, with dedicated care, and yes, indeed, with public money. The script included Dr. Julius Hess, the director of Sarah Morris Children's Hospital at Michael Reese and head of Chicago's Medical Society. Formidable. And Dr. Herman Bundesen, the health commissioner, a man who was known to be mighty fond of the microphone himself.

Plus, this show was going coast to coast, riding on the airwaves out above the dusty plains, the sharecropped farms, the railroad beds, the tenements, the crystal-and-teacup avenues, the shantytowns, the ranches with their cattle stock, the tidy homes and offices, the luncheonettes and smoky joints in all the little cities all across the USA.

For today, the radio host would keep his cool and wipe his brow and hold the laughs in check.

M artin Couney, in his custom quarters—air-conditioned—on the midway, had every conceivable reason to be in a splendid mood. Here came his moment, and could you believe it? Everything he'd ever done was leading up to this. All those years of eminences looking down their noses, as if it were in questionable taste to save a life. Tawdry, they called him. Unscientific. Up to something fishy, just because he'd gotten rich. Not once had he billed the parents of his patients a nickel. No matter what color, religion, or class—penthouse or alley—he'd saved them the same. The audience paid, and if he'd made money, what business was it of anyone else?

They'd tried to shut him down and shut him up. They'd painted him a rogue and a risible figure. Yet several doctors had spent a summer learning from him, a fact they conveniently liked to forget. Only Julius Hess had been his faithful ally, all the way back to those long-ago days in Chicago, both men young and hopeful.

How many babies had gone to their graves? Chicago was one thing, New York was even worse. The rest of the country, forget it. First, they said the incubators didn't make a difference and then they stopped to question if these babies were worth it. It wasn't as if there was any shortage of hungry mouths to feed. Why sweat these small ones, who might be a burden?

Over in the Great Hall within the Hall of Science, the public could view a display explaining eugenics. Propagation of the fittest. Selective human breeding would eliminate the "feeble," the "degenerate," the possibly defective. Also in the hall, the fine men of science were showing pickled fetuses for public edification. And yet, the infant incubators counted as amusement.

Martin was growing old in this endeavor. At sixty-four, he was losing his hair, while his girth had grown thick. For thirty-odd years, he and his wife, Maye, along with Louise—"Madame" to the public—had executed every clever stunt they could concoct to get the press to show up. Every day that no one paid attention was a day that children died.

To hell with the heat. He dressed with Old World elegance, no matter the weather. What he lacked in height, he made up for in comportment. Some might say he should reduce, but where was the need? His work was his life, but a man had to eat. The steam that arose from a redolent plate; the bouquet of a fine, aged wine; and a table filled with guests—there was possibly nothing better than that. Except for a baby.

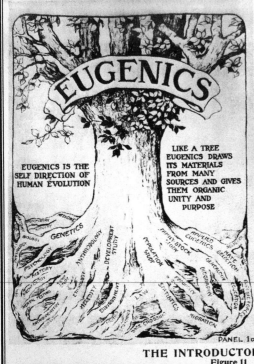

EUGENICS

EUGENICS IS THE SELF DIRECTION OF HUMAN EVOLUTION

LIKE A TREE EUGENICS DRAWS ITS MATERIALS FROM MANY SOURCES AND GIVES THEM ORGANIC UNITY AND PURPOSE

GENETICS

PANEL 1a

WHAT EUGENICS IS ALL ABOUT

Eugenics is that science which studies the inborn qualities – physical, mental and spiritual – in man, with a view to their improvement.

Nothing is more evident in the history of families, communities and nations than that, in the change of individuals from generation to generation, some families, some races, and the people of some nations, improve greatly in physical soundness, in intelligence and in character, industry, leadership, and other qualities which make for human breed improvement; while other racial, national, and family stocks die out – they decline in physical stamina, in intellectual capacity and in moral force.

Both good and bad qualities are hereditary. It follows that every family and every race, as well as every nation, has its own eugenic problems. When the new generation is produced by sound and capable families "the breed of man tends to improve." If, however, the more degenerate members of the community produce the greater number of children, then "the breed of man degenerates."

The eugenical future of your community – and in parallel fashion of your family and your nation – depends upon (a) who moves into your community to become the ancestors of a portion of its future citizens, (b) how the present members of the community – both native and adopted – marry, and (c) how many children the different families have in relation to the "excellence of the hereditary stuff out of which they are made."

Eugenics, then, concerns improvement in the breed of man. Obviously it is closely parallel, in essential nature, to the improvement in domestic plants and animals; but it is clear that in man the methods of mate-selection, and of reproducing from the best and forbidding reproduction by the most inferior, must be different from the methods employed in plant and animal breeding. Applied eugenics works essentially through long-time education, in which young people build up an appreciation of the importance of "blood" and "breed" – that is of the hereditary foundations of individual and family success. In the long run, the appreciation of good blood is counted on to influence mate-selection and family-size ideals – unconsciously perhaps, but just as really and as powerfully as wealth, social position and charming personal qualities.

PANEL 1b

THE INTRODUCTORY PANEL
Figure 11

The eugenics exhibit at the Century of Progress Exposition consisted of a series of four wall panels showing the aims of eugenics as exemplified in human pedigree studies. The first panel was a graphic representation of the relation of eugenics to other sciences and a brief introductory statement.

A baby!

All the world loves a baby—this was his slogan, written at the door to every show. To gauge by the crowds, it was true, at least when Maye made the babies delicious to look at, with ribbons and bows. But no one—not Maye or Louise, not even, perhaps, the parents themselves—appeared to adore a baby more than he did. The light in the eyes, the fragile breath, the cheeks. The initial sparks of cognition. And then the chubby toddlers who were brought back to visit. More recently, the creamy invitations: a high school graduation, the wedding of someone no one but he and Louise and Maye believed would see a single birthday.

Every blistering, footsore day, he would station himself at the door to his show—*All the world loves a baby! Once seen, never forgotten!* He never got tired of talking to the public, not even the *Dummkopfs* who deduced he'd *made* the little critters. (*Hiya, Doc, where'dja get the eggs?*) Sometimes they wanted to order one fresh for themselves.

To terrified parents, he offered reassurance. Maybe their child was the weight of a little undercooked brisket, maybe the obstetrician shook his head. Martin promised life. And sure enough, most of the patients went home in a couple of months, daintily dressed by his wife. Maye, a highly trained R.N., would give instructions (feed every two hours, love all the time). He would proffer a glossy autographed photo of himself, signed "Uncle Martin" or "Your foster father." Louise would sign her likeness "Aunt Louise."

Maye avoided cameras. She tended the babies and kept the books and managed all the rest of it—the nurses, wet nurses, supplies, the business end. She didn't have a word in the radio script, but she would be plenty busy today.

M aye knew this reunion was costing a fortune. Her husband was extravagant—give him a dollar and he would spend three. Today, they were serving an elegant luncheon to more than forty people. Forty-two silver cups had been engraved, to be presented to the babies.

Every day, Martin saw the money coming in at the gate, which was tremendous, but she saw the bills. No expense was spared, no possible corner cut or tucked inside the nursery. And every night, while the Deco lights blazed on the midway, they hosted multiple seatings at dinner, for staff and wet nurses, and always the guests. Medical men who might think twice, and then again, before endorsing her husband in public wouldn't say no to filling their bellies at his table. He'd courted them relentlessly, for all the years she'd known him. Back home in New York, he favored high-end restaurants, but here in Chicago, they rarely left the fairgrounds.

Martin loved to cook. He could make a feast, he said, from nothing—a soup bone. But in his midway kitchen they had plenty more than bones. His palate was discerning: He knew one fancy mustard from the next. These midwestern eaters, raised the way Maye had been, on pork chops and corn, might find themselves developing a hankering for gourmet delectations.

INFANT INCUBATOR COMPANY

NEW YORK WORLD'S FAIR 1940, Inc., FLUSHING, NEW YORK

SOCIETY FOR THE PRESERVATION OF INFANT LIFE

INCORPORATED UNDER THE LAWS OF THE STATE OF NEW YORK

TELEPHONE HAvemeyer 6-8180

AWARDED
GOLD MEDALS

BERLIN,	1896
LONDON,	1897
OMAHA,	1898
PARIS,	1900
BUFFALO,	1901
PORTLAND,	1905
MEXICO CITY,	1908
RIO DeJANEIRO,	1910
SAN FRANCISCO,	1915
CHICAGO,	1933-1934
NEW YORK,	1902-1938
ATLANTIC CITY,	1902-1938

INSTITUTIONS
AND SCIENTIFIC
DEMONSTRATIONS
IN ALL THE
PRINCIPAL CITIES
OF EUROPE
AND AMERICA

May 29, 1940.

May 29, 1940.

My dear Mrs. Ashe:-
    I am enclosing an admission pass for two
people to the New York World's Fair on Friday June 14, the date
of the reunion which I am holding for the babies that secured their
start in life at my Baby Incubators in 1939.
    The pass has been issued in your name for your-
self and one. If your husband is able to accompany you I shall be
very pleased to see him but in event of his not being able to
attend the reunion, you can bring someone with you to assist in the
care of your baby.
    The luncheon for my guests will be served
at I P.M. and the presentation of the cups and the diplomas will
be made after that.
    Looking foward to the pleasure of welcoming you
and your baby, I remain,
            Cordially yours,

            Dr. M. A. Couney

Pass can be used at any gate.

Martin would continue to add to his credentials.

Julius and Clara Hess were often at their table, along with Herman Bundesen, as well as Morris Fishbein, the editor of the peer-reviewed *Journal of the American Medical Association*. Morris liked to bring along his daughter Barbara. That young lady would never forget *les escargots*.

For today's radio program, Martin was going to play it graciously modest. Fluent in French and German, exuberant in English, he could be jolly Uncle Martin, or courtly, or worldly, as needed. Reporters and tablemates swallowed his personal story, which he continued to perfect. Born in France or Germany (depending on who was asking). Often enough, he said Alsace. Matriculated in Berlin and Leipzig, two notably scientific cities. From there, he went to Paris to apprentice with a world-renowned doctor, Pierre-Constant Budin. Yes, his medically educated tablemates had heard of that name.

In 1896, he said, Budin sent his handpicked, German-speaking protégé (that would be himself) to the Great Industrial Exposition of Berlin with the mission of showing a new invention. Budin had developed infant incubators and was using them with great success at Paris Maternité. Young Martin had a vision: Rather than display the incubators vacant, he would demonstrate with living, breathing preemies, borrowed from a German charity ward. He called the exhibit *Kinderbrutanstalt*—"child hatchery"—and before it even opened, it had inspired drinking hall songs. The show itself, he would later say, outdrew the Congo Village and the Tyrolean yodelers.

Enter a British impresario named Samuel Schenkein. This dandy showbiz genius, having seen the child hatchery, invited Martin to Queen Victoria's Diamond Jubilee, to be held in London the following year. Budin gave his blessing, and the show was another smash.

On to another continent. In 1898, Martin made the transatlantic crossing for the world's fair in Omaha, Nebraska. There his story swerved (as if it weren't already strange enough). What motivated him to leave Europe

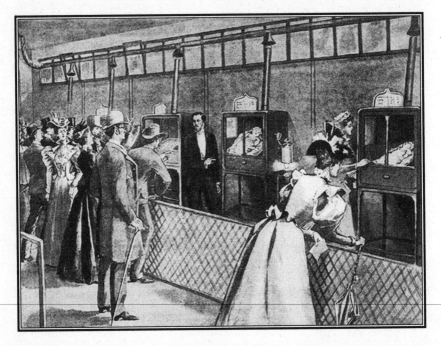

Earl's Court, London.

for good? Once you've seen Omaha, you can never go back to Paris? No one really asked. Assume opportunity. Americans always did. After a quick trip back for the 1900 Exposition Universelle, he bid Paris Maternité adieu, booked passage to the New World, and never looked back. He also never practiced in a hospital again.

Once in a while, Martin's story changed. Occasionally, he said he'd invented the incubators himself. But for today, he would let the other doctors do the talking.

Today and every day, Louise was in the nursery checking her charges. Powder and ointment, diapers and milk, vomit and waste; this was the stuff of her life. And worry. And faith. Every blessed day and all through the night. Was anyone sick? Who was losing ounces? Spitting up? Turning blue? Whose color was ever so slightly off?

One look and she knew, quicker than Martin, quicker than any duckling physician who came to assist him. She and Maye could nourish a child too weak to suckle. No one was better than she at feeding a child through the nose, one tiny drop of breast milk from a wet nurse at a time—hours, days, years of this. She had known Martin longer than Maye had. She had left Paris for him, for this, her American life, holding an

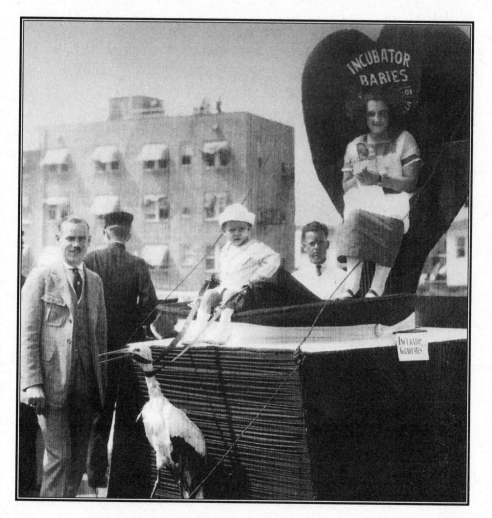

Hildegarde Couney, holding a preemie, atop an Atlantic City float.

infant, fragile in her arms, the ebb and flow of the breath, the whisper-thin skin, the body almost as weightless as the soul itself.

All the hot summers of sideshows and barkers, sharing a home with Martin and Maye; and Maye's widowed mother, until she died; and Martin's cousin Isador; and dear baby Hildegarde, who called her Aunt Louise. Hildegarde was grown now, a nurse like her mother; she was running the show in Atlantic City while her parents were away.

Some days a child was lost—out of sight of the crowd, in the back—the body fevered, undeveloped, no breath in the lungs. At least that little person had been given a chance. So many, Louise knew, would never receive even that. To make the point, you entertained the audience. She gave them "Madame." And she was good at it too.

Martin liked to call it "propaganda for preemies." Whatever it took, she would do.

Not two months back, Martin had lost what might have been the chance of a lifetime to make propaganda. On May 28, a woman in rural Ontario gave birth: one, two, three, four, five. Premature, and how could they not be? Never had anyone heard of five surviving. Triplets were at a tremendous risk—rarely did all three live. Twins were endangered. What could be done about five? William Randolph Hearst had a genius idea: Send the famous Martin Couney!

Martin was a man who lived for *yes*. For once, he said *no*. And in a minute he'd regret it. Yvonne, Annette, Émilie, Cécile, and Marie—the Dionne quintuplets—were now the most famous children on earth. But how could he have known? Having never laid eyes on these girls, he could only surmise that some of them would die. And what if all of them did? The last thing he needed was a public disaster.

No one could fault him for demurring on the grounds that he was already committed to the babies in Chicago. And no one had to guess about what might have been his deeper reluctance—the secret that might leak and put an end to his career.

Today brought another, possibly more important chance of a lifetime. Eleven o'clock in the morning, the mothers began to appear. They came from every corner of Chicagoland, glimmering with sweat, adjusting their loveliest summer frocks, walking in newly polished shoes, while their twins and singles mewled and hollered and spit up and cried like any other toddlers under the blazing sun. Here were Martin and Maye, resplendent and eager to greet them. Here came Miss May Winter, from the class of '01. And here was the always impeccable Julius Hess, and Herman Bundesen, and with them Morris Fishbein. A curious crowd gathered, quite possibly oblivious to the news that halfway around the world, the Nazis were staging a coup in Austria.

At 12:45 p.m. on July 25, 1934, the CBS radio host intoned, "We bring you the world's first Homecoming from the Incubator Station at the Century of Progress in Chicago." He opened by introducing Dr. Martin Couney, who stated, briefly and simply, that at least 85 percent of the babies currently under his care were going to survive. Next, Mrs. Mollie Greenfield expressed her gratitude on behalf of all the mothers of the class of '33. Then the announcer handed the microphone to the city's health commissioner.

"All the world loves a baby," Herman Bundesen began.

THE OBIT THAT WOULDN'T DIE

New York City, 1950

On a Thursday morning in March, an ambitious young doctor was reading *The New York Times* when something caught his eye. Within the decade, William Silverman would be regarded as one of the leading pediatricians in America. He would become director of neonatal intensive care at Babies Hospital of Columbia-Presbyterian in New York, and he would gain a reputation for his insistence on evidence-based medicine—as in, prove it before you use it.

William Silverman came of age in an era when doctors all too often followed their hunches down the path of disaster. In prosperous, postwar, sunny-side-up, baby-booming America, the infant incubator (with its plastic dome modeled on the B-29 bomber) was standard equipment in hospitals. This was the good news. The bad news was the widespread use of treatments that hadn't been clinically tested. One theory held that since two- and three-pound humans can easily die from vomiting and diarrhea, it would be wiser not to feed them at all for the first few days. It worked! No more unwanted effluvia! Unfortunately, the patients died of starvation. Mortality rates shot up, and infants who survived had a higher risk of brain damage. Add "starve a baby" to the scrap heap of abandoned medical practices, along with, say, draining the blood out of someone who's sick.

Another disastrous theory had to do with oxygen. If oxygen helped preemies breathe, the thinking went, then more of it ought to be better. As a result, a generation of infants—among them Stevie Wonder—was going blind because of a mysterious condition called retrolental fibroplasia. Later in the 1950s, William Silverman would be among the doctors to solve the puzzle.

Everyone needs a hobby, and Dr. Silverman's was reading the *New York Times* obituary pages. No day was complete, he wryly told his colleagues, until he found out who'd died. On March 2, 1950, he picked up the paper and saw a most peculiar item, the subject of which was one Martin A. Couney, age eighty. This was a name no one would find in a medical textbook, yet according to the *Times*, the "incubator doctor" had treated preemies for half a century in American amusement parks. Coney Island! Atlantic City! World's fairs! Outrageously, this fellow charged admission to look at his patients. And yet, he had some stellar European credentials. Very odd, indeed.

For a moment, William Silverman thought he had never heard of this man—and then, in the way that memory sometimes lifts the shade an inch—he realized that, yes, in fact, he had. Like millions of other people, he had visited Chicago's Century of Progress in 1933 and, now that he thought of it, he had passed a sideshow advertising living babies in incubators. This was long before the problem of retrolental fibroplasia, before most hospitals even treated babies in incubators, let alone gave them oxygen. The show, he recalled, wasn't in the Hall of Science but out on the throbbing midway. He was only fifteen at the time, but even then, it struck him as bizarre.

Had Martin Couney been alive on March 3, 1950, the meticulously scientific William Silverman might have rung him up. And had the latter been in passable health, he'd doubtlessly have extended an invitation to one of the city's premier dining establishments. We can imagine the scene: The courtly European, well known to the maître d', and the Cleveland-born doctor linger over rare gigot and no few glasses of wine. The room begins to empty for the evening. Martin Couney has cleaned his plate of every delectable morsel, soaking the juices into the final iota of chewy bread. He waxes passionate about saving the tiniest lives, invokes his French mentor—the great Pierre Budin!—and at the mention of his late wife, Maye, sheds a tear into a linen handkerchief, weepily sentimental in old age. He deftly deflects every penetrating question: Exactly which medical school did he attend? Where, precisely, was he born? Why the devil would anyone practice serious medicine on the midway? The wine is of a terrifically pricey vintage. When the second bottle is drained, Martin Couney produces his wallet without so much as a glance at the tab. His guest gets up from the table with more questions than he came with, but this has been a most congenial meeting, and perhaps is the beginning of a lasting friendship.

Alas, as noted in the *Times*, Martin Couney was dead. And now, if such a thought may be indulged, he seemed to be teasing from beyond the grave, playing a game of "Catch me if you can." Who was this tantalizing man, who practiced something akin to vigilante medicine?

Martin Couney published nothing. Untethered by institutional affiliations, he moved in the ephemeral, flash-and-dazzle world of the midway, surrounded by flaneurs who left little but pixie dust behind. Records? It would be easier to track the incubator doctor's gas and electric bills than to gather information about most of the babies who'd spent their earliest days in his care. As for the name Couney, that was neither French nor German. It could have been Irish—if it were spelled "Cooney." Spelled with a *u*, it seemed to trace its roots to the beautiful land of make-believe.

William Silverman, one of the sharpest medical minds of the twentieth century, fully intended to get to the bottom of this. He had no inkling how many years he would spend, and that he would never fully uncover the start of this cockamamie story.

A SHOWMAN IS BORN

Prussia, 1869

In the Prussian town of Krotoschin, a woman cried out in labor. Her name was Fredericke Cohn, and she and her husband, Hermann, had left Alsace-Lorraine just a couple of years ahead of the Franco-Prussian War, as trouble rumbled across the border. Fredericke already had three children—Max, Alfons, Rebecca—born in quick succession. Now she was racked with the pains of labor again. Heaven knew this child would be her last. On December 29, 1869, as the decade ended and a bloody new one was about to begin, Fredericke gave birth to Michael.

Krotoschin (now Krotoszyn, in Poland) holds a contradiction: As with many places in Eastern Europe, its history seeps through its pores at the same time it is hollowed by erasure.

Whatever Hermann Cohn did for a living, the records are lost. But Fredericke's people, the Levys, were doctors. One of their number was said to have ministered to Napoleon himself. Now she was raising her children in a city with little room for advancement. It was home to a well-known publisher, the Bar Loebel Monasch Press, a purveyor of prayer books and a celebrated edition of the Jerusalem Talmud. Among the

Talmud's more famous sayings: If one saves a single life, it is as if one has saved the world.

But most of the assimilated Jews here weren't scholars. They were merchants and small-business men, and before the nineteenth century ended, they would begin to leave, with the population dropping up to and after the Great War.

Only seventeen Jewish people would be left in Krotoschin in September of 1939, when the Nazis rounded them up and deported them to the Łódź ghetto.

But in 1869, the Cohn family, now complete, could not have foreseen what the twentieth century would bring.

ET VOILÀ! THE ARTIFICIAL HEN

Paris, 1878

Nine winters had passed since Michael Cohn's birth. Seven bitter winters since the Franco-Prussian War. The Germans had besieged and starved Paris, and brought her to her knees, and captured her sovereign, who would die in exile. But a renewal had finally come. And with it an Exposition Universelle, staged on the same proud acres as the exposition held before the war. Not since Napoleon III walked these grounds had Paris seen such grandeur. The purpose was to show the world that France was back, her glory undiminished.

Or almost. Alsace had been lost. Both the home the Cohns had left and the town to which they'd removed themselves now belonged to a newly unified Germany. Nevertheless, if the family hadn't moved such a distance, they might have considered visiting this fair, with its clever inventions, its sumptuous gardens, its art. Michael might have delighted in viewing the head of the Statue of Liberty, before she sailed away to meet her body. By working on the armature, an engineer named Gustave Eiffel was building his reputation.

Yet for all the industry, invention, and determination on display, for all the symbolic rebirth, one critical national resource remained in short supply. The literal French birth rate, which had already been declining through the 1860s, was dropping like a guillotine.

Dr. Étienne Tarnier was passing the afternoon at the zoo. Let the rest of the city go to the exposition and sweat it out with the tourists. As the head obstetrician at Paris Maternité, he had other considerations. This population plunge was deeply troubling. When war came again—as everyone knew it would; only a fool would think otherwise—how would there be enough soldiers for France to stand a chance? With too few children, how would the French economy survive? The beloved culture? Who needed enemies when France was poised to murder herself from within?

The edge of the blade was women having fewer children, working outside the home. Not much he could do about that. But the babies they bore were dying all too often. Already, Tarnier had developed axis-traction forceps, a new design that would help with stubborn heads. At fifty, he was making a dent in treating postpartum complications such as puerperal fever. But what about the infants born too soon, too small—the feeble ones, the "weaklings," as they were called in the medical literature? Under 2,000 grams (4.4 pounds), maybe seven months' gestation, they were almost certain to die.

The Jardin d'Acclimatation, the zoo in the Bois de Boulogne, offered plenty to contemplate that day. The place itself had risen from the dead. During the war, besieged Parisians, reduced to consuming any available flesh—equine, canine, feline, rodent—ate the zoo's unfortunate inhabitants, sparing only the monkeys, who looked too unnervingly human. A pair of beloved elephants named Castor and Pollux appeared on the menu of a restaurant called Voisin, in the form of "braised elephant pudding," proof that one might face starvation with panache.

Of late, the zoo had been restocked not only with animals but also with human beings. First, it was Africans and Eskimos, then Argentinian gauchos and "Lapps." In the name of anthropological interest, visitors came to gawp, as if these *others* belonged to a different, inferior species.

Étienne Tarnier was having none of it.

He had come for chickens. Specifically, he wanted to inspect the new machines designed for hatching and fattening them. To watch a chicken peck its way out of its shell is nothing short of mesmerizing: A minute before it was only an orb, now it's a feathered thing, like hope. As Tarnier sat and watched, he was struck by a revelation: If poultry could be nurtured in an incubator, why not premature humans?

At Leipzig Maternity Hospital in Germany, the head obstetrician, fifty-eight-year-old Carl Credé, had already spent more than a decade saving weakling babies using a machine called a *Wärmewanne*. Similar "warming tubs" had been used even earlier in Russia. In these devices, the baby lay on a dry bed surrounded by a double-walled jacket of hot water. Lacking body fat, with sluggish circulation, underdeveloped nervous and respiratory systems, and improper metabolism, a premature infant was liable to freeze to death—especially at a time when "room temperature" in winter might have been 50 degrees Fahrenheit. Peasants would try to save their weakling babies by sticking them inside a jar of feathers. Another remedy was to slather the feeble one in olive oil, wrap it in cotton or sheepskin, set it by the hearth, and hope for the best. Most of the time, the best was not good.

The *Wärmewanne* wasn't perfect. It required constant vigilance. But Credé had made significant advances over years of solid work. And Étienne Tarnier's "epiphany" would irk him.

Carl Credé could tell you where that chicken-loving Frenchman had found his inspiration—and it wasn't the Paris zoo. Tarnier's ambitious intern, Pierre-Constant Budin, had examined the *Wärmewanne* on a recent trip to Moscow. What's more, Tarnier had requested additional information about it from Leipzig right around the time he had his clever poultry moment. Tarnier's proposed contraption was enclosed and Credé's wasn't, but the concept was the same.

This was a point that was hard to dispute. But Carl Credé's rival would publish first.

By 1880, Étienne Tarnier had his *couveuse* (translation: brooding hen) up and cooking at Maternité. To build it, he'd hired Odile Martin, the engineer who had made the chicken hatcheries. Why look farther than you

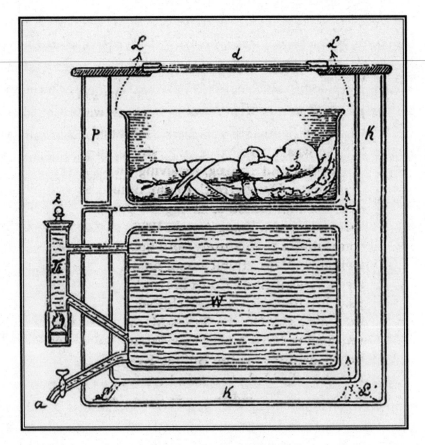

One version of the Tarnier couveuse.

had to? This "artificial hen" was a two-tiered device. The bottom held a reservoir of water, which was heated by an outside boiler called a *thermosiphon*, powered by an alcohol lamp. The upper deck held multiple newborns, poultry style.

Tarnier reported that his *couveuse* cut the mortality rate of weakling infants by half. There was, however, a delicate situation. The *couveuse* was a closer relation to a pressure cooker than to a mother hen. The boiler was so potent and the flow of gas at the charity hospital so uneven that, left unchecked, it raised the possibility of boiling the water in its bowels—and stewing the patients above.

To skirt that gruesome risk, the nurses got in the habit of refilling the reservoir by hand, ditching the *thermosiphon*. Tarnier and another of his interns, Alfred Auvard, set to work retooling the machine. Instead of a reservoir, they used simple hot-water bottles, and they reconceived the upper deck to hold just one baby. By this point, it was not so automatic or impressive.

For his part, Pierre Budin, the man who'd first seen the *Wärmewanne*, must have had it in his mind not to let his fellow intern, Auvard, get too far ahead of him.

WILLIAM SILVERMAN AND
THE COUNEY BUFFS CONVENE

New York City, 1970

D
r. William Silverman stood up to make a speech. The occasion was the Newborn Dinner, an annual gathering of pediatricians held near Atlantic City.

Two decades had passed since the ink had dried on Martin Couney's obituary. At various times over the past twenty years, William Silverman had found people who'd known the incubator doctor, but his inner circle was gone. A couple of medical journals such as *The Lancet* referred to the sideshows, and a few historical archives offered photos. One of Silverman's best finds was Evelyn Lundeen. She'd been the late Julius Hess's head nurse for the run of his career, and had been dispatched (not entirely happily) to help at the Century of Progress. An expert herself, she had published articles and pamphlets on caring for premature infants, and had been honored as Illinois Nurse of the Year.

During an afternoon spent feeding martinis to the elderly Miss Lundeen, Dr. Silverman gathered that she'd found Madame's diamond-ring-over-the-infant's-wrist routine distasteful. Yet she had to concede that the Frenchwoman's care of the preemies had been flawless.

B y now, Dr. Silverman had a few colleagues who shared his fascination. Dr. L. Joseph Butterfield, at Children's Hospital in Denver, having learned that the incubator doctor spent one summer in his city, began to poke around. Dr. Lawrence Gartner, a professor of pediatrics and chief of neonatology at Albert Einstein College of Medicine in New York, discovered that a friend of his mother-in-law's had been Martin Couney's patient at Coney Island; his mother-in-law had seen Baby Gladys in the show.

Drs. Silverman, Gartner, and Butterfield began to call themselves the Couney buffs, and over time, more joined. Lawrence Gartner scoured New York and Atlantic City, looking for anyone who'd been associated with the showman—Gladys, of course, but also doctors, an Atlantic City ambulance driver, mothers of the children. These people strained to capture fraying threads of memory. If only they'd written it down, they said. But even if they had, it wouldn't have mattered. Not even those who'd enjoyed a daily acquaintance knew much about Martin Couney, really. He was friendly. Elegant. The ambulance driver, Jerome Champion, remembered, "He wasn't pretentious, he was real nice to you. He'd say, 'How are you, Champion?'"

T apped to invite the speaker for the 1970 dinner—a festive event, with banquet and cocktails—Lawrence Gartner made the perfect choice.

The room was in high spirits as William Silverman approached the podium. "I've always felt a little bit concerned about the speakers at these neonatology dinners," he began, warming up his audience. "The thought of facing several hundred drunken neonatologists always terrified me."

Already, he had the room laughing. "I remember once I was addressing a pediatric society in Virginia. And there was a very generous cocktail party and a grand dinner. And in the middle of the dinner, a barbershop quartet came in and sang. And everybody was feeling just grand. Then the chairman got up and said, 'Dr. Silverman will now talk about twins!' You can imagine how that went over," he said, to more laughter. "Well, I'm not going to talk about twins today. I'm going to tell you about a story that began, for me, on the second of March, 1950 . . ." He acknowledged that some of them had already heard him speak about his favorite investigation, but the information kept changing.

"Martin Couney was born either on the thirtieth of December in 1870 in Alsace, or on the thirty-first of December, 1860, in Breslau," he said, playing the lack of clarity for humor. "He was educated in Breslau, as near as we're able to find out, and in Berlin, and received his M.D. degree, and then he went to Paris to study with the famous Pierre-Constant Budin. . . ."

Amid the clinking silverware, the atmosphere was one of delighted interest and amusement. Pity next year's speaker. How could anyone top this?

MICHAEL COHN SEES AN ELEPHANT, AND THE LIGHT OF A NEW WORLD

SS *Gellert, 1888*

The passengers boarded at Hamburg, hopeful and wistful and nervy with fear, and already homesick, some of them. The journey to port had been wretched. Rattling on trains from hometowns all throughout Germany. Stopping at inns that robbed them for the privilege of tossing and scratching all night on a bug-infested mattress while thieves stuck sticky fingers in their pockets.

Those bunking in steerage went aboard with their few clothes, their last marks, the warmest blankets they could scrounge, despite its being August. They went clutching their family photographs, their neatly creased letters of recommendation, their handkerchiefs smelling of someone left behind. They brought aboard lemons for seasickness, and rough maps, and wild schemes, and lingering coughs that they tried to suppress.

The New World was their destination, but the old one they were leaving was in a transformative period. In Turin, forty-four-year-old opium-addicted Friedrich Nietzsche would enter his last productive months. The year before, he had completed *On the Genealogy of Morals*, a text that Benito Mussolini would later twist to his own ends. In Silesia, Gregor Mendel was dead, but the seeds of the science of genetics—and reposing within them, eugenics—had been planted. In Arles, Vincent van Gogh was ripping visual paradigms; in a year, he would sever his ear. In Paris, Gustave Eiffel was constructing something exceptional for the next Exposition Universelle. Elsewhere in the City of Light, Étienne Tarnier was tinkering while his interns, former and current, eyed succession. And at the port of Hamburg, an eighteen-year-old from Krotoschin was boarding the *Gellert*, steerage class. His name was Michael Cohn.

Michael would have done well to slip up to the open deck. The berths smelled of vomit, and worse. People were crying. And moaning. Bemoaning. Fourteen heaving, seasick days and nights of this—but soon

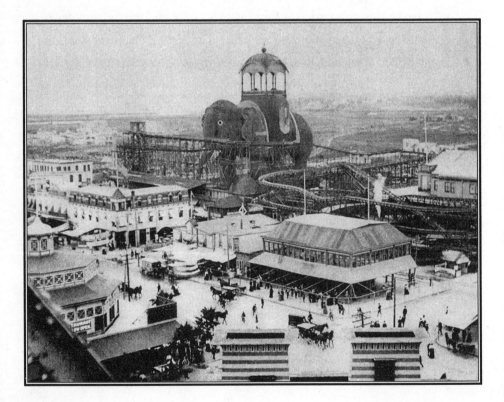

they would be in New York. Michael's mother, Fredericke, would miss him, but surely she knew there was nothing in Krotoschin for him. His father had died. And everyone young was packing up and moving westward, deeper into Germany or crossing the ocean. His brother Alfons emigrated first. He'd left for New York at barely fifteen. Jaunty, stylish Alfons had changed "Cohn" to "Coney," and now he was a jockey at the races, at least when he wasn't working as a clerk at a bank. Whatever the situation, Alfons seemed to finesse it.

The immigrants were eager to see the Statue of Liberty, two years old, holding her torch aloft. But first they were going to see something else. It looked like . . . an artificial elephant? This was Coney Island in the distance. Sodom by the Sea, with its high jinks, its gamblers, its cabarets, its dancing girls, its houses of flagrant ill-repute. Apparently, the people on this island had completely lost their minds. The pachyderm-shaped building was the Elephant Hotel, a seven-story novelty colossus with telescopes embedded in its eyes. Someone from within the beast could have been watching the Germans at that very moment.

The *Gellert* rounded the horn at the base of New York, and the more auspicious sight of Lady Liberty appeared. Magnificent. She could make you cry, this time for joy.

Soon Michael Cohn would stride away from the cloyingly vomitous air of steerage and into the thrillingly filthy oxygen of New York City. First stop, Castle Garden, the immigrant intake center. Someone was going to peer inside his mouth, look down his throat, write down his name. Anything could happen in this strange new country. Alfons must have taken his name from that crazy Coney Island. Perhaps he would do the same, in time. Already, he had made a decision regarding "Michael." Michael didn't suit him. He preferred "Martin." Martin Arthur. Yes, that had a ring to it.

THE COUNEY BUFFS ENCOUNTER
THE MYSTERIOUS M. LION

New York City, 1979

fter twenty-nine years, William Silverman was ready to lay his pet
project to rest. His article about a "colorful (and bizarre!) chapter in
medical history" was set to be published in *Pediatrics*, the peer-
reviewed journal of his profession.

Certainly, William Silverman had more pressing concerns. Increasingly, he worried about the ethical implications of advanced technologies,
of taking extraordinary measures to save barely viable infants who—*if*
they survived, if their deaths weren't being painfully prolonged—might
suffer from catastrophic physical and intellectual disabilities. In the years
ahead, he would publish probing essays under the not-so-secret pseu-
donym Malcontent. He would wonder "whether neonatal medicine's
enormous increase in technical power has allowed it to become coercive."
When is it cruel to force a heart to beat?

That question continues to haunt the beginning of life—as well as its
end. What do we do with the means to keep someone alive in a near-
vegetative state? To what extent does it matter if that someone is an infant
or a nonagenarian? Technology, from life support to genetic testing and

editing, keeps making the choices harder: *Which lives are worth living? Who decides?*

By contrast, this diverting business with the sideshows should have offered satisfaction, an itch well scratched.

In August of 1979, William Silverman's article saw print. He acknowledged a few remaining "loose ends." Nevertheless, this was a comprehensive reckoning, incorporating all the research from his fellow Couney buffs. Paris. Berlin. London. Omaha and Buffalo. New York, of course. Chicago. Photos of the incubator doctor, young and old, spiffy and staid, and later decidedly sad-eyed.

And so the matter was settled. For a minute.

And then the letter arrived in the mail. West German postmark. Its

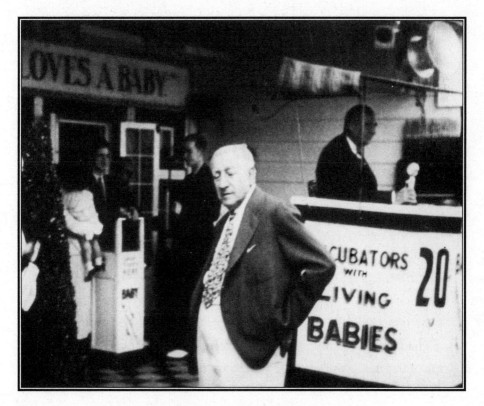

By the late 1930s, Martin had lowered the price of admission.

author, a credible-sounding reader named Felix Marx, begged to differ with a fact about the Industrial Exposition of Berlin. His quarrel wasn't with the "child hatchery" or with the drinking hall songs it spawned. The problem was, the man who brought this show to Berlin was not named Martin Couney. It was someone named Lion.

And with the vibration of that tiny roar, the entire foundation of Martin Couney's story began to fall apart.

"THE GREATEST NOVELTY OF THE AGE!"

London, 1897

What was not to love? London, with its carbonated energy, the babies being saved, the attention Martin and Sam—Messrs. Coney and Schenkein—were receiving with the marvelous invention they were showing! The Diamond Jubilee for Queen Victoria's sixty years on the throne was a wonderland of arts and entertainments, yet they—two American immigrants—were singled out for notice.

This was more than worth the nasty transatlantic crossing. Sam—born in Kraków—had the money and Martin had the charm. Together, they had a winning proposition. Already, these incubator shows were a hit in France. And just last summer in Berlin, the crowd had been ecstatic. More than one hundred thousand people saw the exhibit at the Industrial Exposition. Six thousand women came to look in three days alone.

Messrs. Coney and Schenkein had secured exclusive rights for London for this summer. How could those fellows over at Barnum & Bailey help envying them? But this was not a silly entertainment. It was educational, important. Top-of-the-line: the gleaming machines with their handsome German imprint, the French nurse who knew what to do with the babies, their spot across from the exposition's welcome center at Earl's Court, guaranteeing traffic.

Martin's job was host, shaking hands, greeting guests, answering endless questions. Every day, with something like 3,600 people. The spiel might go like this: *Yes, the tiny babies you are looking at are real. Yes, most of them will live. No, they can't hear you. The heat comes from these coils, you see. It's all automatic. Did you say you're a physician?* Martin was a natural. Diminutive yet stylish, genial yet eloquent in just the right measure. He could talk to anyone, workers with faces ragged from hardship, delicate ladies, men with callused hands, and those who held a surgeon's knife. And they were saving lives! Where Sam saw shillings, Martin saw babies' faces.

The gentlemen at *The Lancet* saw a step in the right direction. On May 29, 1897, before the show even opened, the editors had noted, "The employment of incubators as a means of saving the lives of prematurely born or of very weakly infants has not yet become general in England. Yet it is notorious and obvious that the best, almost the only, means of saving such infants is to protect them absolutely from change of temperature and from cold." In just the past year in England, 2,534 infant deaths had been attributed to prematurity. *The Lancet* mentioned previous inventions, by Carl Credé and Étienne Tarnier, but those machines were extremely difficult to maintain. "The main feature of this new incubator," the editors wrote, "is the fact that it requires no constant and skilled care. It works automatically; both ventilation and heat are maintained without any fluctuations whatsoever, not only for hours, but even for days. The incubator need not be touched for these purposes, and the only attendance necessary is that needed for feeding and washing the infant."

Martin was in no position to disabuse them of that notion. But from where he stood, he must have seen that the feeding (every two hours during the day, with the watchman waking the nurses every three hours at night) and the cleaning (not just bathing the babies but keeping the whole place spotless) mattered as much as the heat. The French nurse, Mlle. Louise Recht, worked harder than he did, sometimes feeding the weakest through the nose with those funneled spoons she had. When anyone asked, he and Sam explained that she was specially trained at Paris Maternité. That commanded respect. They had wet nurses, too, and British physicians checked on the infants daily. But Louise was the person they couldn't do without.

Late at night, after everyone else had left and the grounds had fallen quiet, with only the watchman and the nurses stirring, Martin might have stayed and talked with her, in French. Perhaps it was she, perspiring in the heat of the feeding room, who showed him—the baby of the family—how to hold a newborn.

A cross the channel in France, M. Alexandre Lion was doubtless satisfied by his invention's success, though it couldn't have been a surprise. After Berlin, nobody would have expected anything less. All one had to do was take a look at what passed for competition—the tricky *couveuse*, the clunky *Wärmewanne*. The awkward, wheeled brooder that the American doctor Thomas Morgan Rotch rolled out at Chicago's White City exposition in 1893. Dr. Rotch laid claim to being Harvard University's first professor of pediatrics, but his invention was doomed. Besides the poor design (even aided by a technical expert), the doctor didn't have the wit to display the machines with babies inside. Typical academic.

To build a worthy incubator, you didn't want a professor or a physician. You wanted an engineer. As for Odile Martin from the Paris zoo, he was clearly out of his depth. In the superior system that he, Alexandre Lion, had devised—brilliant, if he said so himself—warm air circulated via a spiral water pipe, heated by a reliable boiler. The thermometer he affixed to the side recorded a constant, ideal temperature. Problem solved. Yet here was another way his invention was better: ventilation. A fan blew fresh air into and out of the incubator, with a pipe that led outside, and a disinfecting filter. His machine was also pretty, with a generous glass window affording an enjoyable view of the baby lying inside. For feedings, the weaklings were taken to a "dining room" and fed by breast, or in the case of those too feeble to suckle from a wet nurse, by tiny drops of breast milk, fed through the nose with a funneled spoon.

With all of this, who needed a hospital? Those were nasty places anyway, hotbeds of infection. In 1891, Lion opened a show in his hometown, Nice. The babies were charity cases, and given the urgent nationalistic need to save them, the municipal government gave him funding. So did the wealthy society ladies who liked to come and look. The public was invited, free of charge. Why not?

Two years in, another genius initiative: host a reunion to prove that his patients—of all races—had thrived. A year after that, he reported saving 137 out of 185 babies, about 74 percent. The only ones he lost, he said, weighed less than two pounds or had mothers who'd waited too long to deliver them into his care.

A doctor was almost superfluous. Parents could buy this and use it at home. Nor did Lion give much credit to his nurses, implying that the primary prerequisite was youth: They had to be capable of staying up all night. He hired them for six-month stints, replaceable pieces of his scheme.

From Nice, he expanded to Lyon, Bordeaux, Marseille, and Paris, where, without government help, he found himself required to charge a modest admission. At the Infant Incubator Charity at No. 26, Boulevard Poissonière, Parisians paid fifty centimes to see babies described by a reporter as "just big enough to put in your pocket." That same reporter stated that "like the bearded lady at the circus," the show was worth the price.

It seemed as if the only person not convinced was Dr. Pierre Budin, the man who'd succeeded in succeeding Étienne Tarnier as the head of obstetrics at Paris Maternité. Budin and Lion moved in different circles, yet the pediatrician decided to give the new machine a try. But the gas supply to the hospital was still so hit-or-miss that even with the much-improved boiler, it was hopeless. Back to hot-water bottles.

In fact, back to the mother. At Maternité, the rudimentary *couveuse* was placed next to the mother's bed to encourage maternal bonding. Breast, breast, breast. In this, Budin was relentless. A leading cause of infant death was diarrhea, and he believed cow's milk was a culprit. He set up clinics to teach new mothers about nutrition and hygiene. He also used *gavage*, Tarnier's system in which infants too weak to suckle were fed through a tube, not with a spoon like Lion's.

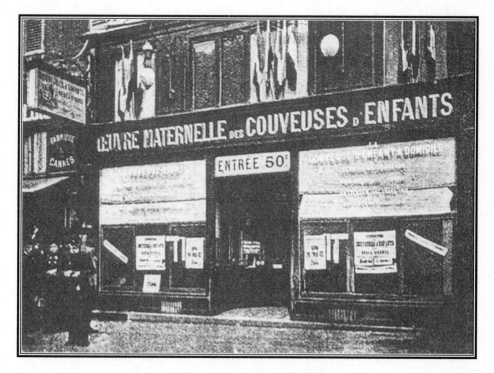

No. 26, Boulevard Poissonière, Paris.

Budin would be dead before the babies he'd painstakingly saved would be summoned to the battlefields of World War I, some of them blown to bits before they were out of adolescence.

Alexandre Lion was strategic. He secured an invitation to the Industrial Exposition, knowing that recognition in Berlin would count for more than whatever he did in France. Before the show's opening in Treptower Park, he applied for a German *Patentschrift* and licensed the instrument maker Paul Altmann to manufacture his invention. Altmann had as solid a reputation as anyone could wish for. His clients included Robert Koch, the physician who'd discovered the bacterium that causes tuberculosis.

On every possible level, the show in Berlin succeeded. The "child hatchery" wowed the crowds, but the official name was the Children's Incubation Institute, and prominent doctors, including the highly regarded public health advocate Rudolf Virchow, gave it their blessing. The Germans wanted to make the exhibition permanent.

Alexandre Lion wanted to go home. Upon his return, *The Lancet* would shower him with praise: "Little children have ever been esteemed the most precious of human possessions all the world over, but it was reserved for an energetic Frenchman to set the seal upon this preciousness by conserving the immature specimens in glass cases." People might visit his Paris show, the journal wrote, "to obtain resolution of their doubts by ocular demonstration."

As for the Germans, Lion said they could keep the machines and proceed without him. And if a pair of American immigrants wanted to license the rights for London, he wouldn't say no to that.

All that summer in London, the press was lit up. "The Greatest Novelty of the Age!" Well, that was a paid listing. But also, this, in a journal called *The Sketch*: "It works automatically, thus dispensing with the necessity for incessant watchfulness." Similar statements were made in the London *Times*.

The articles might as well have said: *Calling all showmen, give it a go!* They couldn't buy from Altmann? How hard could it be to build a copycat contraption? The lines continued to wind around the Americans' concession. You can't upstage a baby.

Or maybe you could. Just get your own and say it was smaller. The casual observer would never know the difference. It wouldn't be long before even the Royal Aquarium was in on the act, as if to suggest, *Fish, babies, it all comes from the same primordial slop, yes?*

M essrs. Coney and Schenkein were not amused by the competition. The letter they sent, written in Martin's signature style, was nothing short of a work of art, all the better for avoiding any mention of M. Lion.

On September 18, with the Jubilee still in swing, *The Lancet* published it.

Sirs,

In the interests of the general public we desire to call your attention to the fact that the success of our Infant Incubator Institution at . . . Earl's Court has attracted the notice of unscrupulous imitators. We are informed, for example, that various persons are calling upon, and writing to, members of the medical profession, hospitals, infirmaries, &c., asking for their support, and falsely representing that they are opening branch institutions in connexion with us, and asking for the loan of children to experiment with.

We consider, under these circumstances, that it is our duty to warn members of the medical profession, also nurses, parents, and all public institutions, not to entrust their children to any applicants whatsoever without first taking every precaution to assure themselves that they will not be made the victims of showmen, as well as of inexperienced and

irresponsible persons who seek to trade upon the established reputation of an
invention that has been recognised by both the medical and the lay press.

The institution at Earl's Court is the first of its kind in England, and we
have not made any arrangements, nor have we given anyone authority to
further exhibit, at any exhibition or place of public resort in the United
Kingdom, so that all persons, no matter what their credentials may seem to
be, making application for space and intimating that they have the power to
exhibit Mr. Paul Altmann's invention should be classed as impostors.

> *We are, Sirs, yours obediently,*
> *Samuel Schenkein*
> *Martin Coney*

Undeterred, the "impostors" kept at it. By February of 1898, *The Lancet's* editors were fed up. While the "favourably noticed" exhibit at Earl's Court was a serious and well-run endeavor, they wrote, "it attracted the attention and cupidity of public showmen, and all sorts of persons, who had no knowledge of the intricate scientific problem involved, started to organise baby incubator shows just as they might have exhibited marionettes, fat women, or any sort of catch-penny monstrosity. It is therefore necessary that we should at once protest that human infirmities do not constitute a fit subject for the public showman to exploit."

Particularly grievous was a show at the Agricultural Hall, Islington: "Just opposite the incubators there are some leopards and everyone is familiar with the obnoxious odor that arises from cages in which such animals are incarcerated. There is a similar exhibit at the Royal Aquarium, and we cannot think that the dust of bicycle racing, the smoking of the men, and the exhalations from the crowd of people who visit that resort are likely to constitute an atmosphere suitable for prematurely born infants. . . . Is it in keeping with the dignity of science that incubators and living babies should be exhibited amidst the aunt-sallies, the merry-go-rounds, the five-legged mule, the wild animals, the clowns, penny peep-shows, and amidst the glare and noise of a vulgar fair?"

Obnoxious leopard odors were the least of it. The editors had finally conceded that the incubators weren't magic ovens. You couldn't just pop in a baby and wait for it to be done. Somebody needed to keep the machines and every inch of the premises immaculate, or lethal disease could spread. Somebody needed near-infinite patience to properly feed the most delicate mammals on earth. And somebody needed to manage rashes and vomit and excrement and everything else that propels itself out of a baby.

A bloody lot of work. London's showmen didn't give a fig about *The Lancet*, but it wouldn't be long before they decided premature infants weren't worth the bother.

Martin and Sam were already back in America, getting ready for their Omaha show. Martin must have believed that a change was in order. Although his brother Alfons was correct—you were better off keeping under your hat the fact that you were Jewish—his name lacked gravitas. Alfons had a knack for finding trouble. Already he'd spent a night in jail for fisticuffs, for breaking a fellow's nose at the Gravesend racetrack, fighting over the books. That sounded in keeping with "Coney." New Yorkers at that time pronounced it "Cooney"—*Cooney Island*. Mellifluous, yes. But Martin, for the work he planned to do, might need to tweak the spelling.

Part Two

SURVIVAL OF THE FITTEST

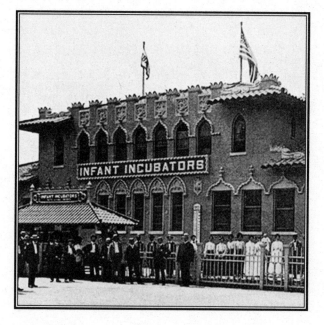

THE MARCH OF
SCIENCE AND INDUSTRY

I n 1933, a twelve-year-old boy took the train from Milwaukee to the Century of Progress in Chicago. His name was Mark Raffel, and he would become my father.

The first I knew of this visit to the fair was almost seventy years later, after his death, when I opened a drawer in his study and found a half-dozen typewritten pages. This turned out to be an "autobiography" that he had written at the age of sixteen. The fair was mentioned almost as an aside, but it piqued my curiosity. I knew there was a world's fair in Chicago in the 1890s. It was famous for its Ferris wheel. But in the 1930s?

T he official 1933 program for the Century of Progress stated: "Individuals, groups, entire races of man fall into step with the slow or swift movement of the march of science and industry."

From the opposite side of the atom bomb and the Holocaust, that notion was disturbing. Unable to let it go, I flew from my home outside New York City to Chicago. There, I spent hours in the History Museum's

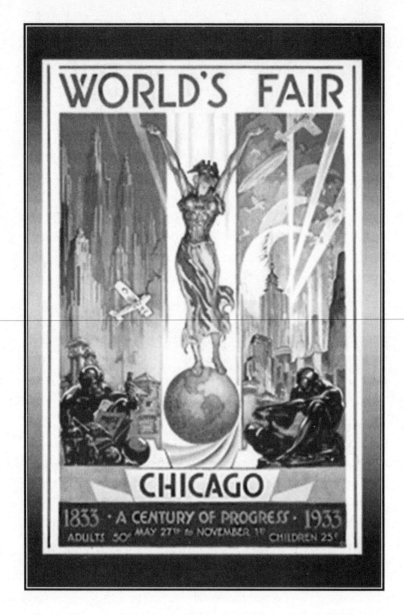

research center, squinting at documents and sifting through photographs. The entire spectacle mesmerized me—science and industry as drivers of humanity. The magnificent Hall of Science, the airplanes and the automobiles, the Enchanted Island of rides for happy children, no few of whom would die in World War II.

But the image I couldn't shake came from the midway: A body-to-body crowd appears in front of a building with the sign "INFANT INCUBA-TORS WITH LIVING BABIES." It seemed to encapsulate everything about this fair: science and industry, married to commerce, bathed in voy-eurism. The future generation as commodity. The doctor in charge was named Martin Arthur Couney, and he had impressive credentials. But who would allow their child to be exhibited in this way? That a proven lifesaving technology existed but wasn't available in most hospitals had never occurred to me, nor was I yet aware of the eugenics exhibit, the real purveyor of babies as product. The incubator show was among the most popular attractions of the entire fair. Even without yet seeing the full pic-ture, it was easy to understand why. Who wouldn't want to view the in-heritors of the Century of Progress baking in their ovens? Given the chance, I'd have done it myself.

B ack home, I stumbled across an item about the Coney Island Museum on Surf Avenue. Years ago, as a young woman transplanted from the Midwest, I'd screamed myself hoarse on the Cyclone, but I lacked the deep connection true New Yorkers have. (One man told me, "I loved Coney Is-land like a person. It had a smiling face.") Still, I thought the museum might give me some insight into early-twentieth-century midways. I per-suaded a friend to join me, and on a bright summer day, we rode the F train underground and up again to its rattling end.

We found the museum across the street from the new Luna Park, with its whirling, lose-your-lunch rides and its whack-a-moles and its paper-cup piña coladas. Upstairs from the museum's first-floor "freak bar" were a couple of rooms full of artifacts from the heyday of America's trippy playground. Photographs and reproductions. Funhouse mirrors. Now you're fat, now you're tall. You've lost all perspective. Something knocked me for a loop. *Coney Island had an incubator sideshow.* This wasn't a special event like the Century of Progress. It lasted forty years, until 1943. How was that even possible? And then I saw the name of the doctor in charge of this thing.

"It's him again!" I told my bewildered friend.

THE ARRIVAL OF THE EMINENT
DR. MARTIN ARTHUR COUNÉY

Omaha, Nebraska, 1898

The gangly man had a hatbox in his hands. "Is the doctor still around?" he asked. Martin was closing up his concession for the day. And this tall man with the workingman's hands appeared to be selling something, whatever was in that box. Martin didn't want to know. "The doctor has left for the night," he said.

Eight a.m., another day beginning, and here was this fellow back, still carrying the hatbox.

Martin had no choice. He had to admit he'd fibbed: *He* was Dr. Counéy. The visitor handed over the box. "Here is a baby my wife had yesterday about twenty miles from here," he said. "I been sitting up with it in the park."

Martin lifted the lid. Sure enough, the hatbox held a tiny baby, still breathing.

But decades would pass before Martin would tell this tale—and add, for good measure, that the baby lived.

The Trans-Mississippi Exposition was nothing like the triumph of London for Martin, or Berlin for Alexandre Lion. Omaha was remote. If anything, this fair aimed to poke Chicago. Its Grand Court was called "The New White City." The original White City—formally, Chicago's Columbian Exposition of 1893—had set a new American standard, with its alabaster Beaux-Arts refinement, its breathtaking Ferris wheel (see that, M. Eiffel?), its hootchy-kootchy dancers and raunchy shenanigans out on the Midway Plaisance. Culture was worthy, but frankly, the midway was where you made money. Back East at Coney Island, George C. Tilyou, heeding the siren song of coins pinging into the till, opened an amusement park named Steeplechase, after the nearby racetrack. Tilyou knew the country's thirst for midway entertainment had scarcely been whetted.

But Omaha was far away from Sodom by the Sea, and no match either for that soot-belching, hog-killing, crime-infested metropolis squatting

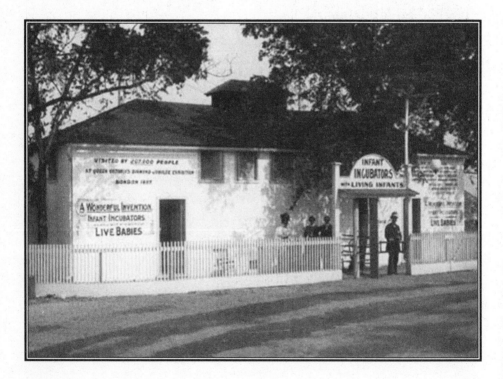

indelicately on Lake Michigan's shore. The Trans-Mississippi Exposition would (in theory) be an affair with nicer manners. No immoral entertainment. No "spirituous liquors" sold. *The Omaha Bee*, on its front page, raved: "To the spectator it would seem that some long forgotten magician had escaped from the dingy covers of an ancient fairy tale and caressed the bare expanse of bluff and stubble with his creative wand."

The president was obliged to show up. Every American world's fair, previous and henceforth, demanded such a visit. Seventy thousand people packed the grounds on October 11 when William McKinley arrived. McKinley had "pushed the button" in Washington, D.C., to formally open the fair on June 1, but now he was here in the flesh. Amid vast quantities of flesh. Malodorous flesh. Can't-see-a-darn-thing flesh. Perhaps only the dignitaries could fully discern the mock battle of Indian braves staged for the president's entertainment. Next up on the program, after the "savages" were paraded past McKinley, came the livestock viewings. Said one local booster: "The gay throngs on the Midway cheered him, the old soldiers called his name in endearing terms, and the journey was one of interest and pleasure, with no single word of discourtesy to mar a day filled with many pleasant events."

Martin's incubator station sat on the East Midway, not far from the Wild West Show and the camel ride and the Mammoth Whale and the German Village, where presumably he could get something decent to eat. His modest white building looked sleepy. The signs exclaiming "WONDERFUL INVENTION" and "Visited by 207,000 People at Queen Victoria's Diamond Jubilee" seemed almost to be pleading.

Reporters ignored him. Perhaps his operation was diminished without the exceptional Mlle. Louise. The infants on display might not have been as tiny, by necessity, and possibly that hurt him at the gate.

Whatever the explanation, the arrival from France of the eminent Dr.

Martin Arthur Counéy attracted less notice than, say, the naked French painting in the art pavilion. Before the fair, the latter incited an angry man to fling a chair through the canvas. Repaired, the life-size nude—*The Return of Spring* by William-Adolphe Bouguereau—drew many new lovers of art.

Alexandre Lion had enjoyed a more solicitous American reception the previous autumn. The show he opened at 2 West Eighteenth Street in Manhattan was greeted with approval, but he had no intention of staying in that godforsaken city.

His heart was in France. He left his New York setup in the hands of a physician, where it quietly fizzled.

Martin was reduced to hawking beer. "Dr. Martin Couney says nursing mothers cannot find its equal as a milk producer. It is also beneficial to the babes," the ads read. (The accent *aigu* he'd added to his name would prove to be a nonstarter in American newspapers.) Plus, Dr. Couney—"who has had a wide experience"—claims, "We take pleasure in stating we have used Krug Cabinet bottled Beer constantly and for milk producing qualities we can cheerfully recommend it to all nursing mothers." Well, that was one way to get his name in the papers. People said that drinking beer was good for nursing mothers—but still, this was undignified. The next fair, in Buffalo, would have to be better.

As Omaha wound down, Martin had one last piece of business. On November 3, 1898, he stood in the district court of Douglas County, raised his hand, and swore an honest oath. Sam was his witness. Exiting the courthouse, Mr. Martin A. *Coney* was an American citizen.

NAILING JELLY TO THE WALL:
THE COUNEY BUFFS GAIN A FOLLOWER

I left Coney Island determined to find out whatever I could about Martin Couney—a search that quickly led to William Silverman's article in *Pediatrics*. I found another item, about the letter from Felix Marx raising the issue of M. Lion. After that, the Couney buffs had one last piece of business in the pages of the journal. William Silverman's letter to the editor, published in 1997, was cosigned by eleven colleagues. Under the header "Martin Couney's Story Revisited: Writing History Is Like Trying to Nail Jelly to the Wall," he reported more exasperating discrepancies in the showman's story and concluded, "We write this letter to your readers in the hope that others will come forth with additional information about this curious episode in the history of newborn medicine."

Reading it more than a decade later, I hoped that William Silverman was still alive somewhere. That would have been highly unlikely. His *New York Times* obituary ran under the headline "William A. Silverman, 87, Dies; Leading Neonatologist of 1950's." It was published on January 2, 2005. Too bad he couldn't enjoy it over his morning coffee. And too bad I hadn't tried to reach him sooner.

"THE PRESIDENT HAS BEEN SHOT!"

Buffalo, New York, 1901

The new American Century was born to the sounds of the horn and drum and stomp and clap of John Philip Sousa's marching bands, to the mischievous syncopation of Scott Joplin's ragtime, to the heat and spice of a million immigrant kitchens. In England, Queen Victoria entered her final month of life. In America, William McKinley wouldn't outlive her by much.

M. Alexandre Lion had returned to France to stay. On April 14, 1900, another Paris Universelle Exposition began, with its Art Nouveau and its talking films and its latest great invention—escalators! And yes, an infant incubator exhibition. M. Lion printed copious souvenir postcards with his likeness as *directeur-fondateur*.

On April 10, four days before the Paris exposition opened, Martin Coney signed a business agreement with Samuel Schenkein. Here was a name for you: Qbata. *Cue-BAY-tah*. As in, *Come see the babies in the incubay-tah, dahlink*. This was their new company. With Alexandre Lion gone, Martin and Sam were going to make a grand showing of it. The Kny-Scheerer company in New York manufactured Lion's machines for the

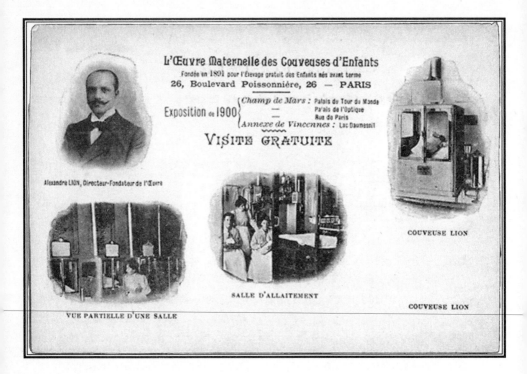

L'Œuvre Maternelle des Couveuses d'Enfants
Fondée en 1891 pour l'Élevage gratuit des Enfants nés avant terme
26, Boulevard Poissonnière, 26 — PARIS

Exposition de 1900 { Champ de Mars : Palais du Tour du Monde
— Palais de l'Optique
— Rue de Paris
Annexe de Vincennes : Lac Daumesnil }

VISITE GRATUITE

Alexandre LION, Directeur-Fondateur de l'Œuvre

COUVEUSE LION

COUVEUSE LION

SALLE D'ALLAITEMENT

VUE PARTIELLE D'UNE SALLE

United States, and a handful of hospitals bought them, including Chicago Lying-in, Low Maternity in Brooklyn, and Sloane Maternity in Manhattan. Copycat contraptions, some of them homemade, and some based on the clearly inferior *Wärmewanne*, were being tried as well. It was bupkis, when you thought of it, and nothing to match the grand showing the Qbata company planned. First on the agenda was the Pan-American Exposition in Buffalo. Next would be Topeka, and then the crown jewel: the Louisiana Purchase Exposition, scheduled for St. Louis in 1904.

The immediate challenge was money. Machines were but a fraction of Sam's projected expenses. Now he needed architects and carpenters. No more sleepy buildings. This would need to be a dazzler. Every world's fair was all but strangled with red tape, which meant he could count on paying workers overtime to be ready on opening day. Plus gas, water, light.

The new electric bulbs that everybody wanted. Blankets, bottles, diapers, powders, tiny clothes and tiny hats, and pink and blue ribbons. Salaries for nurses, wet nurses. Someone to take tickets. A barker to haul in the crowds, which was something you needed out East. The fair's administration would of course require payment. And finally, the cost of demolition. He was going to build a miniature hospital, only to knock it down.

Sam found an investor, Emmett W. McConnell, who would get 50 percent of the gate in Buffalo until his debt was paid, and 25 percent thereafter. Plus, McConnell would take a cut of any profit made from licensing baby powders and lotions—which seemed like a sweet idea at the time.

McConnell was Sam's problem, but Martin had his own. For starters, after Omaha, it might have occurred to him that "Counéy" didn't work. Was it possibly too foreign? Not friendly enough? He would try "Dr. Coney." More than anything else, he needed to find a nurse as competent and self-assured as Mlle. Louise, who was back in France.

Someone recommended Miss Annabelle Maye Segner. Maye (as she preferred) was all-American, raised in Lafayette, Indiana. She had received a bachelor's degree from Indiana University and trained as a registered nurse at Maurice Porter Memorial, a children's hospital in Chicago. And she was thoroughly lovely, with flowing golden curls, the favorite child of her widowed mother.

Maye must have found him charming. Imagine: This Dr. Martin Coney didn't have a clue what to do with a newborn—in fact, she might need to remind him how to properly hold one. But he seemed to care. He was courtly and European, easy to talk to. And while some of the city's physicians would check in from time to time, *she* would run the nursery.

At twenty-five, Maye could have seen her future and not liked the way it looked. Spinster. Dreary halls of overcrowded hospitals that were never entirely clean. Doctors snapping orders, even when she knew more about a particular patient than they did. Every day, growing more invisible. Trapped.

Well, here was her adventure. When Dr. Coney offered her the job, she said yes.

Stately and ornate, at the junction of the midway and the busy pedestrian mall, the infant incubator building would have been difficult to bypass. But just in case, a barker hollered: *Don't forget to see the babies!* Inside, all commotion yielded to peace and common sense. Eight machines stood tall against the walls, while cordons kept the line in perfect order. The floors were clean enough to lick. Miss Maye Segner had taken charge, never revealing an ankle, a forearm, the slightest hint of skin below the collar of her starched white dress.

As soon as a child arrived, she gave it a bath in "synized" water and mustard. If it could swallow, two drops of brandy went into its mouth, and then it was rubbed with alcohol, swaddled tight, given a pink or blue

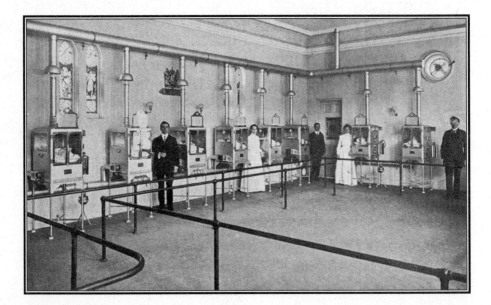

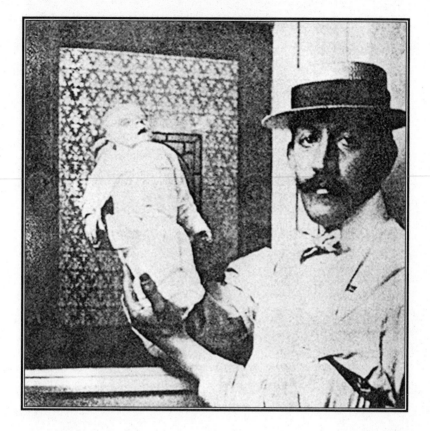

ribbon, and placed in an incubator kept at 96 or so degrees, depending on the patient. And, oh yes, the baby was given a show name, for confidentiality's sake. Every two hours, those who could suckle were carried upstairs on a tiny elevator and fed by breast by wet nurses who lived in the building. The rest got the funneled spoon.

Greeting every guest was Dr. Martin Arthur Coney, with a garter on his sleeve and a bow tie at his neck and a fine, curled mustache and atop his head an Edwardian boater. He lavished attention on physicians, who'd gotten free season passes from Sam, signed "Dr. Schenkein."

Some of Coney's women visitors favored Little Willie, two pounds, fourteen ounces, delivered into the world by a Buffalo doctor. The twin girls were cuties. The baby boy, A.S., as they called him, arrived in bad condition; they were treating an infection in his eyes. To everyone's delight, triplets arrived with their mother on the train from New York City.

Photographers materialized. Martin would pose an infant, its delicate life in his hands. No syllable of worry crossed his lips. Yet his eyes, in the moment when the shutter was released, looked solemn, almost grave, as if he had some inkling of the decades ahead.

Trouble broke out at the Indian Congress exhibition. Cries. A gasp. Apache princess Ikishupaw had gone into labor. The father was Chief Many Tales. In the heat of July, the baby was born too soon—but an incubator awaited!

Was it a boy or a girl? The papers never said. "It" tipped the scales at two pounds, two ounces. *The Buffalo News* declared "it" the smallest child ever born—a compelling statistic, if not necessarily true.

Martin just kept winning with the reporters. They may have ignored him in Omaha, but here in Buffalo they loved him, even the medical journals. *Pediatrics* judged the exhibit instructive, despite its location in an area "almost wholly given over to the amusement of those frivolously inclined." The magazine noted the 85 percent survival rate (without any clinical evidence) and further stated, "The exhibit is one of, if not the most popular, in all the Midway."

Scientific American repeated the 85 percent survival rate. Ordinarily only about 25 percent of infants born "prematurely or weakly" lived. "Most of the babies lie with their eyes closed, and practically the only sign of life is the occasional flutter of one of the tiny hands."

Arthur Brisbane, among the nation's most influential journalists, skipped the specifics, waxing ecstatic in the pages of *Cosmopolitan*. The two features of the world's fair most worth seeing, he opined, were "two vast extremes. The weakest and the most powerful manifestation of nature's power. The falls of Niagara, with the great system of rivers and lakes

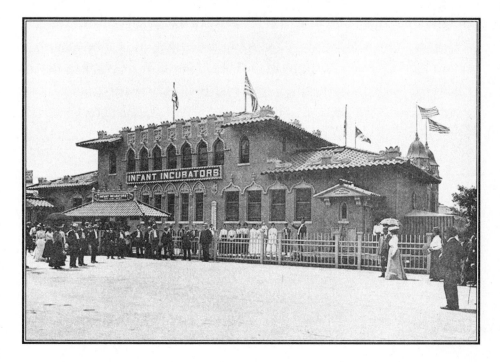

behind them. The diminutive baby in its hot-air chamber, sightless, deaf, feeble—but with the great human race, the vast sea of organized thought back of it." For Brisbane, the babies won the contest. "There is more to interest in the little form behind the incubator glass than in all the roaring and power of 'the Thunder of Waters.'" Further, "The incubator baby begins life in the blissful state of Nirvana, for which the Buddhist struggles through existence."

But one report was chilling. Whoever wrote it didn't sign it. "The question naturally presents itself as to whether this is worthwhile; whether the race as a whole does not suffer from the preservation of these weaklings to perpetuate their kind," the article printed in the *Buffalo Medical Journal* stated. "Medical science is a little illogical in respect to the results obtained, and in its efforts to preserve the individual it forgets to consider the effects of such action upon the race as a whole. Every stock raiser appreciates the necessity of healthful environment, abundant food and fresh air in maintaining a breed of animals in a state of high physical development; and sanitary science insists upon the necessity of these conditions for the physical uplifting of the human race. The stock raise [sic], however, breeds only from the most sound, healthy and perfect animals, and thus secures a physical conformation and constitution upon which the conditions of environment can act most advantageously. Medical science, on the other hand, does not hesitate to undo the advantages gained by the hygienic rules it has promulgated, by preserving the weakling, the deformed, and the tuberculous, and placing these defectives—who would otherwise surely have perished in an active struggle for existence—in a condition to transmit their deficiencies, deformities and vices to generations as yet unborn."

This strain of eugenic thought would cast a shadow over the perception of premature infants and dim their prospects for decades to come.

Dr. Matthew D. Mann was in possession of a fistful of complimentary passes, as befitted a person of his standing. A senior gynecologist and obstetrician at the University of Buffalo, he was someone for whom the term "pillar of society" might have been coined. Son of a senator. Frequently seen on a dais. Active in the Laymen's Missionary League. Past president of the American Gynecological Society and, by the way, an expert in abdominal surgery. As a matter of course, he preserved clippings about his many civic and medical accolades, menus from gala dinners at which he was the honoree, and similar mementos.

Naturally, Dr. Mann had been present among the invited VIPs on the opening day of the world's fair. Along with his season tickets to Darkest Africa and the Indian Congress was the pass for himself and a guest to the Qbata company's interesting show. Colleagues of his apparently were sending their patients to these fellows.

Matthew D. Mann would save his season tickets for his scrapbook.

And naturally, when Mr. McKinley arrived for his presidential visit, Dr. Mann, as a local dignitary, would surely have keepsakes from that.

From the thick of the midway, a trio of showmen was watching Dr. Coney. Damned if this clever foreigner wasn't the same "eminent Dr. Counéy" they'd last seen hawking beer in Omaha.

Frederic Thompson didn't have any reason to pay him much mind back then. He was too busy making money hand over fist. A former architecture student from Irontown, Ohio, Thompson became so smitten by showbiz that he'd taken a gig as a janitor at Chicago's White City, just to find a way in. He ended up getting to run a concession. Five summers later, in Omaha, he presented his own creation. The Mystic Garden was a fantastical cyclorama, a visceral 360-degree vision of heaven and hell. It was the hit of the midway.

The man who despised this show was the son of a prominent Omaha judge. He wasn't morally offended; he was jealous. Elmer Dundy had recently ditched a budding—he thought boring—career in law to chase his jittery bliss. In 1898 he, too, was running a cyclorama on the Trans-Mississippi midway. His was called Darkness and Dawn, and by whatever quirk of the American psyche, his was also a trip though heaven and hell. The difference was, his sat gathering prairie dust while everyone bought tickets for the Mystic Garden.

By the time the afterlife purveyors arrived in Buffalo, they'd had a revelation. Thompson's creativity was out of this world, no way to compete with that. But Dundy understood money and how to play connections. Here was the equation: Genius plus prowess would equal exponentially more than the sum of two individual talents.

In 1901, the former rivals were now partners running several concessions, including Darkness and Dawn (Dundy's name but Thompson's design: "The visitor witnesses the punishment meted out to scandal-mongers, umbrella borrowers and other offenders.") But the big hit was Thompson's latest flight of fancy, A Trip to the Moon. A dime would blast you into outer space, via sound effects and the most thrilling, lift-you-up-off-the-ground electronic engineering anyone had witnessed.

Already, Thompson and Dundy were plotting future schemes. And as they looked around, the partners couldn't help noticing that the baby-saving show was quite the draw, at least as attractive as a ride or a freak.

Elsewhere on the midway, one Edward M. Bayliss of St. Louis was running grand-scale spectacles. His métier was dramatic reenactments of fires and wars, sanitized catastrophes for public enjoyment. In Omaha, the Battle of Manila was a victory for him. In Buffalo, he went for double, with a theatrical production called The Land of the Midnight Sun, using the new electric lighting, and The Great Fire at Dawson City.

Bayliss's shows were highly labor-intensive. In the heat of the summer, he must have wondered why that fake French doctor, or whatever he was, should have a monopoly on a concession that, frankly, looked simpler than staging a disaster.

September 5, 1901, was designated belated President's Day at the Buffalo World's Fair. William McKinley had originally planned to visit on June 13, but the trip was rescheduled when his wife, Ida, fell ill. Now that the couple was finally in Buffalo, the president faced two hectic days. On September 5 he rode the Great Gorge Railway at Niagara Falls, reviewed troops at the fair's twelve-thousand-seat stadium, posed in front of the government building, and gave the requisite speech. "Expositions are the timekeepers of progress," he stated. "They record the world's advancement. They stimulate the energy, enterprise, and intellect of the people; and quicken human genius."

The crowd that afternoon was fifty thousand thick, straining to hear, cramping their necks. One of them had come to kill the president. His name was Leon Czolgosz. And damn this smelly throng, he was stuck, trigger finger itching, too far away to get a reliable shot. That evening, McKinley and his wife, unaware of the near-assassination, toured the grounds in a carriage. Later, the electrical tower was kindled and fireworks rang through the air.

Leon Czolgosz's mother might have told him: Tomorrow is another day.

On September 6, McKinley arrived at the fair's Renaissance-style Temple of Music. His secretary, George B. Courtelyou, thought it a bad idea to shake the public's hands, given the previous summer's assassination of King Umberto I of Italy and an earlier attempt on King Edward VII when he was still Prince of Wales. Courtelyou had tried twice to cancel the press-the-flesh but McKinley wouldn't listen. That morning, as the president met with citizens who'd jammed the building (three thousand inside and another ten thousand outside), Czolgosz waited, gun in his handkerchief. Patience. These adulating tourists. This slow-moving line. Finally, William McKinley extended his hand, his flesh and blood, his pulse. Czolgosz shot him, twice.

The crowd tore into the gunman. They likely would have pummeled him to death had the wounded president not called out, "Be easy with him, boys." He asked that somebody break the news gently to Ida, who wasn't with him, before he was lifted onto a stretcher and carried off.

Everyone was in the streets. To reach the emergency medical center, the ambulance had to pass directly in front of the incubator station, which was in the same square.

News flew on breath, and it stank. Dr. Roswell Park, the exposition's medical director, was out of town, performing surgery in Niagara Falls. In his stead, the center was staffed with junior doctors and medical students. Telephones were ringing all throughout the town. *Answer, answer.* Martin, so close yet so bereft of credentials, was helpless. *If only.*

Inside the medical center, as Buffalo's physicians began to arrive, morphine was administered to cloud McKinley's pain. Dr. Roswell Park was already en route. But as the minutes passed, the team on-site realized they had no time left to wait.

Matthew D. Mann, the obstetrician, was the senior-most surgeon present. He was a resoundingly confident man, but the pressure on him was immense. The doors to the operating theater snapped shut. Burly Secret Service agents stood outside, guns at the ready. They soft-stepped and whispered as "the blood of the Republic" spilled under the surgeon's knife.

Dr. Mann had five other doctors, two medical students, and six nurses attending. But his expertise was extracting babies, not bullets, and he couldn't find the second one. Just the day before, McKinley had lauded the world's advancements on display. Among these was the X-ray machine that thousands of visitors had viewed. By year's end, the first Nobel Prize in Physics would go to Wilhelm Röntgen for the science that made it possible to see through skin and into the body's hidden places. *If only, if only.* Nobody felt competent to use this new invention on the president. Dr. Park arrived just as the operation was ending; the wound was carefully stitched, the bullet still inside. Then the doors parted, first from the operating room, then to the street, where a silent crowd witnessed McKinley being carried out, conscious, on a stretcher.

Terrible things can happen anywhere: Everybody knows it. But here it was in front of them, a lovely day turned bloody. To the immigrant, to the baby nurse, to every man and woman standing sickened in the street, the day would mark the start of an "after."

At first, McKinley seemed to rally. Optimistic updates went out daily from the private residence where the president convalesced. Then gangrene set in. On September 14, his last reported words were, "It's God's way. His will be done. Good-bye, all good-bye."

With that, Theodore Roosevelt became the twenty-sixth president of the United States.

O n October 29, the president's assassin, Leon Czolgosz, was executed. On November 2, the Buffalo fair officially ended.

On November 11, Samuel Schenkein was arrested and the incubators, some still occupied, were seized. "BABIES MAY DIE," screamed one headline. Another reported that city hall circles were agitated by a question about whether Deputy Sheriff Michael Burke was babysitting: He was in charge of "inventory." Included in the seizure were 20 bottles of lotion, 10 dozen infants' linen, 12 dozen toilet powder, 20 dozen toilet soap, 12 dozen jars of toilet cream, 20 dozen tubes of toilet cream, "kindred articles of an estimated value of $1000," and $55 in cash.

The infant incubator exhibit had impressed the public, the press, and much of the medical establishment. Financially, it flopped. Now that the fair was over, the Qbata company's investor, Emmett W. McConnell, was incensed. He sued Schenkein and Coney as involuntary bankrupts, claiming that he was owed $17,250 in receipts, and that his duplicitous partners were hiding assets, which they planned to ferret out of town to the next world's fair, in St. Louis. This last part especially infuriated him: He demanded another $75,000 in damages because they had dealt him out of their plans.

Samuel Schenkein coughed up $1,000 bail; in time, a judge would vacate the order of arrest. Sheriff Mike also caught a break: The confiscated inventory didn't include live infants. They were sent home, with no further word as to their well-being.

The legal and financial mess, however, was only beginning. Buffalo

Children's Hospital bought a few machines, bringing in some cash, but plans for St. Louis were falling apart. Forget about Topeka. Their lotion-licensing business was over before it began. Messrs. Schenkein and Coney, and with them, Miss Maye Segner, were very close to being permanently out of business.

WELCOME TO THE CITY OF THE DEAD

The directions are easy. On a sweltering day, take the J train outbound through Brooklyn. Go underground and up again, past Cleveland and Norwood and Crescent streets, with the life of the city unfolding below. Get off at Cypress Hills.

Proceed along a long and curving road, past rows and rows of graves on rolling land. Some are adorned with flowers slowly wilting in the heat, some with ripening oranges, there to sweeten the passage to the afterlife, some with portraits of the dead etched into stone.

Underneath an underpass, then down a dirt stretch, you will come upon an abbey. Around the back, the door is unlocked. Enter. In a minute or two, your eyes will adjust. Thin light filters in through stained-glass sheaves and holly. A nondenominational chapel waits, vacant. There is birdsong in the distance, if you listen, and a lawn mower's drone. Persian rugs, slightly rucked, will threaten to trip you.

The dead line the walls in rows of drawers, an archive of bones. Up a flight, the light is weaker. Arrows point to famous remains: showgirl Mae West, boxer James John Corbett, steakhouse master Peter Luger. Each notable crypt is marked by a placard on the floor. A former Polish prime minister is memorialized by a bust in a glass case inscribed, "His heart rested here."

Up another flight the darkness is almost impenetrable. Slowly, shapes emerge. A round banquette, like something out of a Hollywood musical dream hotel. Wooden tables for two with aging silk bouquets, and ornate chairs with fabric slightly threadbare to the touch, as if the dead might slip out for a spot of tea, or something stronger.

At the mouth of row LLL, in the bottom-most drawer, alongside his wife, lies Dr. Martin A. Couney.

What did I think I would find here? For months, I'd felt like I was after one of those particles physicists confirm only by the disturbance of their wake. I could have told William Silverman that Martin Couney came from a town called Krotoschin, not Alsace or Breslau. But his census records, starting in 1910, were full of inconsistencies: He was German, he was French, he arrived here in 1884 (at the age of fourteen) or in 1888 (still not possible, I thought), his name was spelled "Coursey," his daughter, Hildegarde, was listed as his wife. Some of these mistakes were clerical errors, others were probably fibs. Hildegarde had disappeared completely. Martin Couney's immigration record was missing and so was the record of his naturalization. The New York State medical licensing archive had no information on him. Between "Coney" and "Couney" and the fact that his funeral had been held at Kirschenbaum's Westminster Chapel, one of the city's oldest Jewish funeral homes, I figured he'd been born Cohen, or maybe Cohn, or Coen, or possibly Kohn, which certainly narrowed it down.

Then there were the babies. In the American Academy of Pediatrics Archives, outside Chicago, among the Couney buffs' papers, I found two letters written by a man named Harold S. Musselwhite, Jr. The first was addressed to "Research Librarian" at the New York Public Library on Fifth Avenue. Dated Thursday, June 27, 1996, it began, "Re: Martin Couney, M.D. I was one of his charges in 1921. . . . I shall appreciate a copy of any obituary record you may have printed and additional information you may be able to provide." What answer he got is unknown, but a second letter, addressed to L. Joseph Butterfield, M.D., was also on file. This one was dated Saturday, June 6, 1998, and it contained a more detailed account of his life. He stated that he was born at home in Brooklyn on April 24, 1921. "My parents and several others were preparing to go to the Statue of Liberty when my mother paused to go to the bathroom. She suddenly called out, 'The baby's here' and I was saved from going down the toilet. . . . It was my maternal grandmother who conceived the idea of keeping me in a cotton-filled shoebox placed in a warm oven as a makeshift 'incubator' until they made contact with Dr. Couney. No hospital had the means to care for me," he wrote. "The 'how' and 'when' is unknown to me as was my means of transportation to Coney Island. Unfortunately, all persons concerned are now deceased and most of the records destroyed." He recalled being told that at his baptism he had "a head so small that it fitted into a small teacup." Mostly he was seeking information, but he wanted to leave a record, too. He wrote about meeting his wife, about his service in the navy, his jobs in insurance and real estate, and the miniature and dollhouse shows he and his wife ran in Mystic, Connecticut. The couple had three children and seven grandchildren. Yet there was something missing: He had never met another of Martin Couney's patients, and yearned to know: *Who else is out there?* The last record of Harold Musselwhite in the pediatric archive noted his website, circa 2001, through which he hoped to find incubator-mates.

After I left Chicago, I found the website—still live, with no evidence of other Couney babies found—and an obituary for Harold Musselwhite, Jr., dated 2005. He'd died at the age of eighty-three, about six weeks after William Silverman. I also found an address for his daughter Joy. I thought she might want to have copies of her father's letters, so I put them in the mail. When she called, she was slightly stunned; her father had never told her some of those things. She didn't know anything more than I did about Dr. Couney, and as far as she could tell, her father had never met anyone else who'd been the incubator doctor's patient.

Some of Martin Couney's patients have to be alive. Almost as soon as I had the thought, an article popped up about sisters named Jane Umbarger and Jean Harrison. The "incubator twins" from the Century of Progress had toasted their eightieth birthday with margaritas at a family picnic in Illinois. A photograph showed the two women wearing flowing summer tops, one pink and white and the other blue and green.

What felt like a minute later, I was on the phone. Jane had the flat midwestern accent of my childhood. For all that I craved information, Jane craved it more. She had wondered for most of her life about Martin Couney. "Was Coney Island named for him?" she asked. "Can you believe they didn't allow him in hospitals?" She and her sister had never met anyone else who'd been in the sideshow, despite living all of their lives in or near Chicago. Her sister Jean had tried writing to media outlets, with no success, although someone unsavory wrote to her once from a prison. More than anything else, Jane wanted to know, "Is there anyone else like us?"

Jane and Jean were born on August 17, 1934, three weeks after the homecoming at the Century of Progress. Together, they weighed seven pounds, ten ounces, which would have been perfect if they had been one person. Their aunt, a nurse, got them into the show.

Every day, Jane said, their father stopped at the fair on the way to his job at First National Bank. He would pass the naughty Streets of Paris and deliver his wife's breast milk to the nursery next door. Among the visitors was a four-year-old boy who would become Jean's husband.

Nineteen years later, strangers crowded the church for the sisters' double wedding. The public had seen them struggle to live, and now—the Depression over, the war won—they wanted to watch the girls walk down the aisle to their happily-ever-after ending.

The second time I called, I had both women on the line. Jean's voice was deeper (she was fifteen minutes older), but the sisters sounded remarkably alike—mid-twentieth-century chipper. Often they said "Oh!" in unison.

"We'd always assumed we were in the Science Hall," Jean said. "We were in our forties or so when we went to an exposition that showed all of the world's fair. And we were on the midway! Like a freak show! We were so shocked to find out." But that shock was amused: a funny midlife treat, like a surprise in a Christmas stocking.

Once again, Jane peppered me with questions: *Was Martin Couney married?* "Oh!" *How long did he live?* "Oh!" *Had I found any other twins? And how did I get involved with this story, anyway?* "Oh, for heaven's sake!"

Jean was still married to the boy whose parents had paid a quarter for him to see her in the incubator.

"Was it love at first sight?" I asked.

"With *my* husband, it was," Jane said. "When he met me, he told his friend, 'That's the girl I'm going to marry.' But I'm not married to my first husband. I've been married to this one for fifty-three years."

I congratulated her, and she said, "When Jean and I got married, I think we were too young. I think because Jean was going to get married, I thought I needed to get married, too, that we needed to have a double wedding." When she met her second husband, they both had two kids already. They adopted each other's children and together they had two more. All those years, both of them worked in her husband's boat-building business. "I'm retired now," she said. "At eighty-one, I think I should be. But I put a lot of years in. You know, it was very busy. Besides raising the six kids."

"That's a lot," I said.

"It wasn't easy," Jane said. "But it's our life." She said it with affection, and yet, almost as if afraid of sounding ungrateful, she quickly added, "I'm happy that I found my second husband, believe me." Jane had lost a daughter eleven years earlier but had fourteen grandchildren and eleven great-grandchildren.

Jean and her husband of sixty-two years—the man who'd glimpsed his future at the Century of Progress—had raised three sons while she worked first at her family's pottery business, then at a newspaper. The couple had nine grandchildren and were expecting their twelfth great-grandchild.

"We hope we're still here when your book comes out," Jane said before we hung up.

I sent letter after letter, hoping I'd found the right address for people whose names had been in a newspaper half a century earlier. I looked up obituaries and sought out the children. *By any chance was your mother in an incubator . . . ?* or *I think this might have been your relative.* People whose parents had been in Martin Couney's machines knew little about the circumstances but told me things like *My mother had a wonderful life. My mother had ten children. My father lived into his eighties.*

Whenever I found a "baby" still alive, she (and it was always *she*) was itching to talk. Each woman, now in her seventies, eighties, or nineties, was tickled that people had paid admission to see her. Each, like Jane and Jean, had more questions for me than I for her. And each was yearning to know, *Who was that man who saved me?*

Welcome to the City of the Dead

In Cypress Hills, I had come to what, in a cruel pun, was another dead end in my quest. I stood there and stood there, staring at the name carved into marble. *Come on, Martin A. Couney,* I willed him. *Talk to me.*

The cemetery prohibits photographing graves, but the man I was visiting wasn't exactly a stickler for rules. And I hadn't seen a living human being since before I'd walked under the underpass. I pulled out my iPhone and took a snap. Later, I saw how dark that photo is, revealing nothing.

TWO ELEPHANTS, A WEDDING, AND A BUNCH OF CRYING BABIES

On Sunday, January 4, 1903, a crowd of invited guests gathered to witness a public execution. Although plans to charge admission had been scuttled, a nervy carnival atmosphere prevailed, with curiosity seekers watching from nearby rooftops, squinting in the winter light. Condemned to die was a healthy circus elephant named Topsy. The men who had ordered her death were Frederic Thompson and Elmer Dundy. The masterminds of A Trip to the Moon were building their own amusement park, visibly under construction. On their orders, Topsy was to be fed arsenic-laced carrots, wired up, and electrocuted with more than 6,000 volts.

Branded a "bad" elephant, Topsy had spent her life being prodded with hooks between her eyes, struck with a pitchfork, and hit with hot pokers, all in the interest of entertaining a circus audience. A few years earlier, a drunkard stuck a lit cigar on the tip of her trunk. She threw him off, killing him. After that, she'd been sold to Sea Lion Park in Coney Island, which Thompson and Dundy had recently acquired.

Topsy's luck—such as it was—ran out when her trainer, Whitney Ault, went on a bender and rode her down Surf Avenue. The stunt resulted in Ault's getting canned, but no one else could handle the three-ton animal. Thompson insisted he tried to give her away but couldn't find a taker. No zoo or circus wanted her, he said. And once he decided Topsy would die, the showman figured he might as well make a buck.

Thompson's initial plan was to have Topsy publicly hanged and charge a quarter admission. Horrified, the American Society for the Prevention of Cruelty to Animals thwarted both the hanging and the profit. But the organization permitted the combination of poisoning/strangling/electrocution, which would be quicker and, they believed, less cruel. For educational purposes, the Edison Manufacturing movie company was on hand to film the event so that Americans nationwide could view it, while Thompson took the opportunity to advertise his soon-to-open theme park.

Topsy refused to cooperate. She wouldn't set foot on the killing platform. Unable to get the elephant to budge, Thompson summoned her old trainer. Ault provided a piece of his mind: He wouldn't coax Topsy to her death. Not for the twenty-five dollars they offered him. The executioners prevailed, moving the platform to where the elephant stood. Into her moist mouth went the poisoned carrots. Next, the electric current ripped through her body. Topsy's wild heart stopped its beating almost instantly, although she was strangled just to make sure. A doctor pronounced her dead.

Samuel Schenkein was back from the brink of extinction. After months of judicial hair-splitting over the nature of Schenkein and Coney's contract with McConnell, the latter saw some cash, but there is no remaining record of how much. Regardless, the cloud of "involuntary bankruptcy" was lifted.

Sam, presumably feeling lucky, bought a ticket. But not for himself. On April 27, who should arrive aboard *La Gascogne* but Mlle. Louise Recht, dark-haired to Maye's golden, now calling herself a more mature "Madame." For the record, she was Amelie Louise, but she, like Annabelle Maye, favored her middle name.

Not three weeks after Louise's arrival, on May 16, Frederic Thompson and Elmer Dundy officially lit up Luna Park, with its half million electric lights and A Trip to the Moon as its signature ride. Roughly a block from the spot where Topsy collapsed, Dr. Martin Couney opened his infant incubator station.

"Come this way, ladies and gentlemen!" the barker hollered. "See the tiniest bits of humanity! Maybe the future president is inside!"

Fifteen years had passed since Michael Cohn beheld the Elephant Hotel from aboard the *Gellert*. A bad idea from the start, the beast became a brothel, until even the hookers checked out. In 1896, it burned to the ground.

Where Coney Island was once a restless nest of vice, now it was a drunk-on-adrenaline fantasyland. Stars and swains arrived in fine, high style. The middle class unbuttoned. Immigrants who suffocated through the week in tenements and sweatshops looked forward to the weekend, when they could cram into airless trains and trolleys, to frolic in the crowded sea. They sunned on the anything-goes beach, surrendering their hard-earned coins at George C. Tilyou's Steeplechase Park. They screamed. They spun on rides that flung them into one another's arms. Lovers slid through dark canals in boats, stealing kisses. Fires raged and wars were won in full-scale reenactments, someone else's hell.

Tilyou's only competition came from the floundering Sea Lion Park across the way. Regardless, he had to keep his theme park peppy. In 1901,

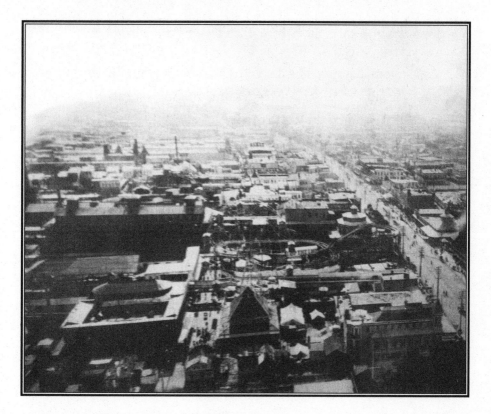

Coney Island from the air.

ever alert for the next best thing, he went on a shopping expedition to the Buffalo World's Fair. He *needed* A Trip to the Moon. And if, in order to get it, he had to hire Thompson and Dundy, so be it. He brought in the partners to manage their hit concession, along with all of Steeplechase Park for the summer of '02. By the end of the season, Sea Lion Park was belly-up.

Tilyou didn't like that. He believed that two parks, like two heads, were better than one. If the neighboring space became a decrepit ruin it would hurt him in the pocket. But he had an idea (he always did). He drew up a cunning second-year contract for Thompson and Dundy that drastically slashed their pay. As he predicted, they stepped right into his setup, huffing that rather than sign this demeaning agreement, they would buy Sea Lion Park instead. So there.

Poor doomed Topsy was forced to haul the mammoth Trip to the Moon to its new location during her final months on earth. The spot where they killed her was less than a five-minute walk from the decomposing ashes of the Elephant Hotel.

r. Coney" had to go. That name would not do. Not in Luna-tic Park, with its lions and tigers and midgets and freaks and blazing lights and strolling bands intended to rouse people up off the benches and onto their swelling feet. A whole Venetian city arose, complete with gondolas; already there was talk of chariots and prancing horses. How was a doctor to run a serious operation in this carnival atmosphere? Certainly not as Coney Island's Dr. Coney. That distinguishing *u* was back for a return engagement—Couney, minus the nuisance accent *aigu* atop the *e*.

"Strangest Place on Earth for Human Tots to Be Fed, Nursed and Cared For," *The Brooklyn Eagle* reported, struggling to contain a paradox in the space of a newspaper column. The idea of "haranguing the passing throng in an effort to divert its shekels for a spectacle so serious, not to say sacred, strikes one as questionable, almost repellent." But then the reporter's assessment took a U-turn, praising the superior equipment, the skillful feeding with the tapered spoon invented by Dr. Martin Couney, and the immaculate conditions, right down to that fact that instead of feather bedding, which absorbed saliva and sour milk, the babies' pillows were filled with a tarred sanitizing substance that was regularly discarded. Indeed, the reporter concluded, this was a "sober, scientific exhibit."

Martin and Maye and Louise might well have assumed it wouldn't be long before every physician and hospital adopted this new system. For now, they could enjoy their good fortune: making money, saving lives, inhaling the ocean breeze.

A lfons Coney would've enjoyed this endearing turn of events. Doubtless he'd have visited, if he hadn't been three thousand miles away, after leaving the Gravesend racetrack for the opposite coast. While Baby Brother saved the babies, Alfons was making a name for himself in certain muscular circles. The following summer, perhaps a bit pickled, he dared a fellow member of the San Francisco Olympic Club to race him up Mount Tamalpais and back to the Dipsea Inn for additional liquid refreshment. Alfons finished second out of two. Nevertheless, he was credited with starting a long-distance-running tradition. The annual Dipsea Race would still be run long after he and his brother were dead and the twentieth century ended.

M artin had lost the coveted chance to exhibit at the upcoming St. Louis World's Fair, but he had gained a home. And now he was going to have a wife. On September 26, 1903, he and Annabelle Maye signed their marriage license, with her widowed mother, Mary Isabella, as their witness. "Belle," as she often called herself, would live with the newlyweds, as would Louise. A family of women. For his marriage license, the city clerk required him to state his profession. He might have hesitated a moment before saying "medical instruments."

He gave his legal name as Martin A. Couney. And this was the truth, or would be in a moment. On October 1, his change of name was finalized by the Supreme Court of the State of New York. Michael Cohn, Martin Cohn, and Martin Coney had gone the way of the Elephant Hotel.

KISS THE BABY

In the photo I found, he looks tired. His hair is mostly gone. His cheeks have fallen into jowls. His eyes, behind black glasses, contain a quiet sorrow. He faces straight into the camera, holding a child so small that his liver-spotted hand covers her torso. The child was named Beth Bernstein and she was born in 1941, the summer before the United States entered World War II.

At birth, Beth Bernstein weighed one pound, ten ounces.

At seventy-three, Beth Allen was petite, almost gamine, with short, straight gray hair and a lively gait. What I saw in her eyes was delight. Martin Couney was clearly among her favorite topics of conversation.

As we sat at her table, with its sweeping view of playing fields and the city beyond, Beth began by telling me about her twin, who lived two days. "I never knew there was another baby until I was about eleven years old and I overheard something at a family gathering," she said. "When I asked my father he said, 'Yes, but don't talk to your mother about it, it's too painful for her.'"

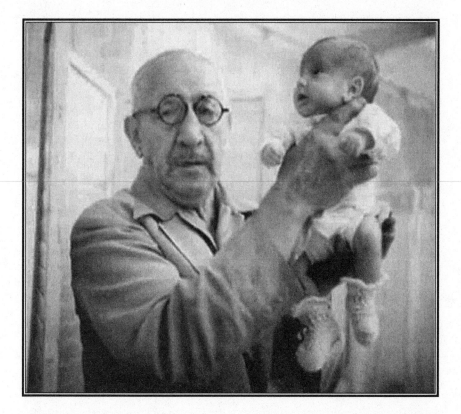

Beth had no other siblings. "I was overprotected all through my child-hood," she said. "When I was ready to come home from the incubator, my mother was terrified. She wanted a baby nurse, but Martin Couney told her, 'No, you've had a long vacation. Now you take care of your child.' She was so afraid that my father gave me my first bath."

If Beth's mother didn't want to discuss her lost twin, she didn't want to talk about Coney Island, either. As strange as that sounded to me, parents *not talking about it* would come up repeatedly as I started finding Martin Couney's few surviving patients. Before I read too much into that, I had to remind myself that theirs was a generation far less fond of "sharing" than ours. Nobody would have spoken openly about a miscarriage, either. No-body talked about illness—certainly not cancer, and nothing connected to intimate parts of the body or the psyche. So much of that past has vanished due to silence. How much of our own past, I wondered, will be lost amid too much noise?

Ten years ago, maybe more, someone named Dr. Lawrence Gartner had wanted to interview Beth's mother. She finally agreed, but the meeting was canceled when his travel plans changed. Instead, he sent Beth a list of questions to ask on his behalf.

"Here's the little piece of paper that I used when I interviewed my mother," Beth said. She had cut the questions short when they became too painful, but now she referred to her few existing notes. "My mother was at her mother's house with one of her sisters when she went into labor," she read. "They called the doctor, who said it must have been something she ate. And her sister said, 'No, no, no, you come over right away.'"

Ah, how often did I hear about doctors thinking labor pains were simple indigestion? But this doctor, persuaded, came over and drove Beth's mother to the hospital. Israel Zion (now Maimonides Medical Center) had a few incubators, but no one there was trained in treating a baby under two pounds. And the hospital didn't have enough machines to keep a single baby for long, when other babies were waiting.

"The doctors wanted to send me to Dr. Couney, and my mother rejected that totally. She said, 'My baby is not a freak. I don't want her in a sideshow.'" Convinced that her daughter had no chance regardless, she was persuaded only when the elderly Martin Couney came in person to plead his case.

Having said yes, she couldn't bear to visit. But Beth's cousins, eleven and eight years old, were full of questions. "The eight-year-old remembered her mother trying to describe how small I was," Beth said. "She took out a pound and a half of chop meat and said, 'This is your new cousin.' The eleven-year-old went to Coney Island every day."

This latter cousin, Terry Silverman, had died by the time I met Beth, but years earlier, she had made a recording for the Coney Island Oral History Project. In a raspy, nostalgia-soaked voice, she spoke about going to see the incubators free of charge, about Martin Couney patting her on the head and about befriending the midgets next door. She also recalled people criticizing Beth's mother: "A lot of people expressed horror . . . 'How could you do that? Put your child on display like a freak?' She said, 'No, my child is being saved by a genius of a man with incubators.'" For all that Beth's mother was embarrassed at Coney Island, she was clearly grateful.

Toward the end of the season, when Beth's weight topped five pounds, she was moved to a beribboned bassinette. "She was the star of the show," Terry Silverman said adoringly, "and Dr. Couney himself placed her in my arms. I felt faint, I was so excited."

Martin Couney encouraged hugging and kissing. His give-them-love

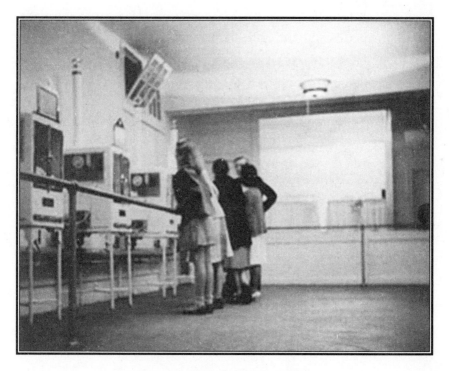

Beth's cousin Terry observes the incubator.

approach was the opposite of the masked and gloved, sterile, *no touch* protocol that hospitals would later adopt—and then reject.

M ore than any of the other "babies" I would eventually meet, Beth had immersed herself in research. She knew that her birth weight remains on the cusp of viability. "When you think of the state of care all those years ago ... I didn't get the blindness, or the lung problems, or the breathing problems," she said. "Now I can't even *lose* a pound and a half."

For Father's Day, her parents would take her to Martin Couney's house by the ocean, visits she barely remembers. "I was a little girl and he was an old man, and I probably didn't want to go," she said. Her parents attended his funeral, but she didn't have any details. "You know, it's just so sad that I never got more information before everyone who lived through it left."

As I was getting ready to leave, Beth mentioned Dr. Gartner one more time. For some reason, the name didn't register with me. Still, I made a note to myself to find this Dr. Gartner—eventually. First, I wanted to do some more digging of my own.

"THE CRIME OF THE DECADE"

St. Louis, 1904

John Philip Sousa's marching band kicked off the Louisiana Purchase Exposition, colloquially known as the St. Louis World's Fair. Innovation like percussion. The ice cream cone, a portable sphere of pleasure you could lick to the final crunch. Mustardy hot dogs and hamburgers. Fizzy Dr Pepper. The midway, called the Pike, looked as if it had sprung from a tipsy pixie's head. Fun and games and rides and freaks and sugar and spice. Visitors could view indigenous peoples—this time a tribe of Igorrotes from the Philippines—and lighten their wallets in all the ways people had come to expect. Left unsaid, hushed up as much as possible in the interest of profit and image: the babies turning blue and dying in the incubator sideshow.

Dr. Martin Couney wasn't there. He and Sam had expanded to Atlantic City, with the assistance of local doctors. Coney Island boasted twin attractions: one in Luna Park and the other in the newly opened Dreamland. Owned by a Tammany Hall–connected businessman named

William H. Reynolds, Dreamland was intended as the lifted-pinkie answer to Luna Park and Steeplechase. Pearl-white buildings, classy pizzazz.
But Reynolds had no showbiz in his veins. In it only for the money, he
copied from Thompson and Tilyou, betting on more being more: If Luna
Park had five hundred thousand electric bulbs, he would have one million.
If Luna Park's Fire and Flames featured a thousand men dousing a confla-
gration, his neighboring inferno would engage two thousand. A ballroom
jutting into the ocean! Three hundred midgets! Preemies!

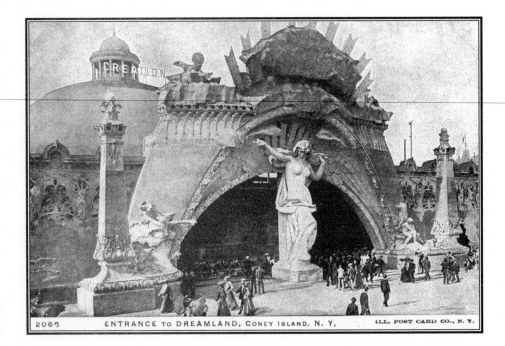

2065   ENTRANCE TO DREAMLAND, CONEY ISLAND. N. Y,   ILL. POST CARD CO., N. Y.

Martin obliged him. On August 1, he ripped a page from Alexandre
Lion's playbook and threw his first reunion. Oh, how he delighted in these
squeezable tots! The triplets from Buffalo, happy and fat. Three sets of
Brooklyn twins, and singles as young as three months old, almost all assured of surviving, thanks to his system.

Later that month, one-pound, eight-ounce Baby Lillian was delivered to the premises. Martin put on an optimistic face and dialed the press. Under the headline "New York Excited over the Smallest Living Body," a reporter remarked that Lillian's fingers were the size of matchsticks.

"The case of Lillian is, of course, the most wonderful in medical science," Martin said, "as no child born weighing less than twenty-four ounces ever has been known to live. I think, however, that she will get along finely now and that we will be able to point with pride to her as a fully grown young woman in a few years."

If only he could speak a kinder truth into power. No further word about Baby Lillian was published, which seems to bespeak her death. For years after, he kept trying to break the two-pound barrier. But Martin's reputation was growing, with plans for concessions in two amusement parks in Chicago, another in Minneapolis (for which he would "train" the personnel), and the Lewis and Clark Exposition to be held in Portland, Oregon, in '05. The future looked as peachy as a healthy child's cheek.

But by the end of the season, the smell of the news oozing out of St. Louis would make Martin Couney sick.

M artin saw it coming. He had warned them, had he not? Never would something like this have happened on his watch. Sam had been invited to make their pitch for the concession in St. Louis all the way back in '01, before their Buffalo troubles. By 1902, the concessions committee was sold on the idea of an incubator show. But rather than award the contract to people who knew how to run it, they were shopping around. For all Martin knew, they intended to give it to Edward Bayliss from the beginning. The master of disaster: the Battle of Manila, the Great Fire at Dawson City. Bayliss was local to St. Louis, well connected.

Still, in the down-and-out December of '02, Martin, as Dr. Coney, was invited to state his case in person. Round and round they went, these men of the committee. The topic was money. Apparently, they were unaware of the lawsuit with McConnell. Sam had offered a flat fee of $8,000 for the concession, while the committee insisted on a percentage of the gate. They refused to relent.

In their meeting with Martin, he declined to reveal financials, either through ignorance or through willful obfuscation. The conversation bordered on contentious, like a bad Mad Hatter party.

"I don't see why it is that you have any objection to stating what your receipts were in Buffalo . . . and I think you take an arbitrary stand."

"Oh, no. It isn't," Martin said. "We have been to a good many Expositions with our affair. We were in Omaha, Buffalo, and Berlin in 1896."

"You were not in Paris?"

At this point he was honest: "No."

"Why not?"

"We couldn't get space."

"Why don't you answer the question about money?"

"Showmen have tried to get into this affair, and we feel it would be wrong to say what this affair can take in, because it would give them, as it were, a line on what this proposition could do. We think it will be a success in St. Louis, not alone from the ethical point of view, but we will make a success of it financially."

"We are not prepared to accept your simple statement. . . . We don't know whether the thing is profitable or unprofitable, other than what you say that, 'It was quite profitable at Buffalo.'"

"We considered it was profitable, because of a great number of concessions in Buffalo that were a failure," he said. "We were able to pay for the installing, pay for the running expenses, and still have a little money to divide among those concerned in it."

"The relative comparison, we cannot understand what you mean by this statement."

"When we saw the failures of others I think we did well. Under our method of operation the affair is placed in charge of your Medical Board and then it goes into the hands of the physicians of the city. When we receive a child, we don't know where it comes from, it may come from a hospital or from a wealthy family. . . . When it is ready to be discharged, the physician is notified."

"How many deaths did you have in Buffalo?"

"We saved eighty-five percent. If we have a child for seven days in our charge we never lose it if it lives that long. Most of the cases we lose as a rule we lose within twenty-four or forty-eight hours after we receive it. The reason for that is that a child of that nature is subject to bronchial trouble, and if we receive it in time, by placing it in the apparatus and keeping it at the proper temperature we overcome that."

Apparently, the committee was tired of talking about the welfare of the children. They shifted the conversation abruptly.

"Are we to understand that your application is withdrawn?"

"Oh, no. You don't want to lose this as a feature of the Exposition."

"It doesn't seem to be what we want."

"We have grown grey in this matter, we have spent many years of our life with this affair in Expositions, and I know you don't want to miss having this as a feature of your Exposition. That is what it is going to be."

"This Committee decided at the beginning that any concession . . . will have to be paid for on the basis of a percentage, not as a fixed sum."

"I want you to consider this as not a simple show concession."

"We regard it as such."

"You ask any of our physicians how they would regard one of your uniformed men standing at the gate of our concession taking a percentage of the gross receipts."

"While we desire the approval of the Medical World, and do not wish to antagonize them, we feel that we have a proposition before us that does not pertain to them, and we must decide upon what lines it will meet with our approval and not how the Medical Profession is going to like it. If you think it is a medical affair, take it to the Medical Department; but we don't think it is."

At last, they dismissed him, but the interrogation wasn't done. John Dunnavant came next. He was there to make his bid for Over and Under the Sea. Martin knew him from Buffalo. The committee wanted John's opinion of Schenkein and Coney. He mentioned "a little difficulty" with the investor McConnell, but mainly he praised them. "There is no question but what they will fix it up right and run it absolutely so that it has the sanction of every physician in the country, and I don't think you could deal with better people to take a thing of that kind," he said.

To no avail.

On January 22, 1903, Sam made another desperate pitch, but he wouldn't bend the flat fee. The committee ended up taking bids from seven concessionaires, among them Mrs. Hattie McCall Travis, who was hoping to run both an incubator show and a daily bullfight, and their former investor Emmett McConnell himself. By August, Sam blinked, offering 25 percent of the gate. But Bayliss, the man with a hand inside, had partnered with a local physician named Joseph Hardy and bested them all, promising 40 to 50 percent, depending on receipts. While he was at it, he made a successful bid for an amusement called the Magic Whirlpool.

Edward M. Bayliss must have wondered why it had taken so long to wrap this up. Now that he'd won, he had no intention of laying a finger on an infant, nor did he plan to stand around shaking grubby hands and indulging ridiculous questions. He would design an ornamented building, turn it over to Hardy, and tune his ear to the beautiful sound of money rushing in.

Joseph Hardy was fully licensed and apparently utterly ignorant of how to care for a preemie. Bayliss, to his credit, purchased Lion-type machines. They were still being manufactured, but doctors were turning against them. With too few specially trained nurses and what little staff they had stretched thin, it was hard to reap the benefits.

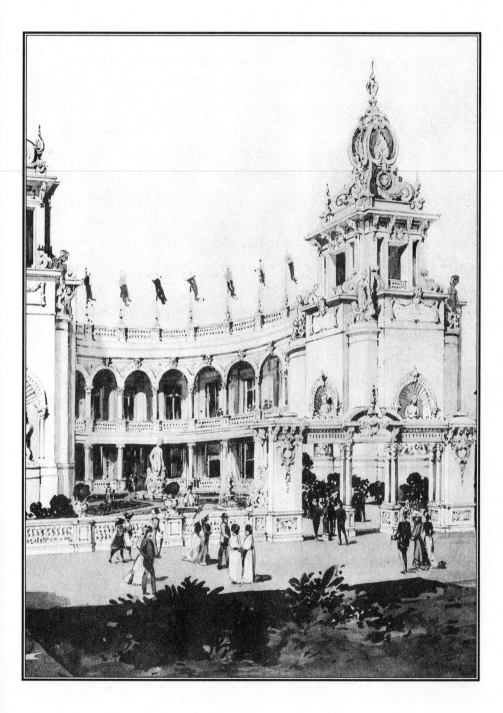

Hardy wasn't worried. To start with, many of his patients were orphans. No parents to breathe down his neck. Once the show opened and word got out, mothers and fathers started calling from all over town for an ambulance to take their newborn to the concession; others boarded trains with their day-old preemies. Most often, the babies died en route. As for the rest, their parents would need to be grateful for whatever help they got. The public ate it up. And the committee licked their lips.

The first child to die had been sick on arrival. Not Hardy's fault. Another baby followed, and another, and another. Infected. In the muggy Missouri summer, machines were overheating. Perfect petri dishes, with no one competent to make adjustments. Plus, Hardy fed the patients cow's milk, not breast, and it soured with contamination. As the body count rose, the good doctor up and quit.

Clearly, this was not the spectacle Bayliss and his cronies had in mind. In the beginning of August, with a young physician hired more out of desperation than for any qualifications, the committee sought the opinions of other medical practitioners. One doctor who had been sending orphans to the show expressed confidence that nothing was the matter: "I have never at any time had reason to think that the place was not admirably conducted," he wrote. In view of the sharply different assessment of others, the question arises as to whether he was enjoying a kickback. A second doctor cited "serious objections," including the fact that the babies were given sunbaths two feet away from "garbage boxes filled with filth."

The most damning report listed dangerously hot machines, poor ventilation, flies buzzing freely, and worse. "The feeding of the babies betrayed the grossest ignorance. . . . For instance, cereal foods and egg albumen were being used for these infants, although it is well known that they cannot assimilate such foods." This letter was signed "City of St. Louis, Health Department."

Still the show went on. The babies kept dying.

A scathing letter, dated September 17, 1904, was sent to the fair's president, David R. Francis:

Dear Sir,

The Humane Society has been investigating the condition of the show at the World's Fair known as the "Infant Incubator." Our officers have made a quiet investigation in the last few days, and we found that everything that has been said about this "show" was and is the truth. We found that for ten days this "morgue" was run without any medical attendance whatever. That the [new] Doctor in charge, O'Neill by name, graduated last May and that since he took charge he has issued about 19 death certificates. That between August 8th and August 19th, '04, ten deaths were reported from this place. Now I want to say to you that the Humane Society is going to press this matter to the full extent of the law, and unless this "Charnel House" is closed at once I will send the officers of this Society out there and close this place by force. This must be done within 24 hours after you receive this letter. I also intend to submit the facts in the case to the Circuit Attorney of St. Louis and also to the Attorney General. Now Mr. Francis if you will see that this place is closed and closed at once there will be no further trouble but if it is not then we will see that it is and the people responsible for the horrible conditions that exist at this place must suffer the consequences. Since this place has been running they have had 43 babies and 39 have died. What do you think of that for a "scientific exhibition." There can be and there is no doubt about the character of this place and that the babies are deliberately murdered through neglect and carelessness, and it must be stopped at any price no matter who has money in this show.

I wish you would give this matter your personal attention and give me an immediate reply so that I may know what further steps to take in this matter.

Yours very truly,
(signed) Rozier G. Meigs

On September 19, a response went out to Rozier Meigs, written on behalf of President Francis, "who is unable to take time for an immediate reply." The fair's management contended that the allegations "come as a complete surprise" and that, with some recent improvements, all was now perfectly well and good at the infant incubators.

Martin, getting wind of it, was livid. Had he not pleaded with the committee to view the treatment of premature infants as a medical matter, not just a money machine? Now he took aim with his weapon of choice. His open letter in the *New York Evening Journal* was prefaced with an editor's note commending it to David Francis, adding for good measure: "It is horrible to think of these delicate babies shut up in carelessly overheated compartments, exposed to the flies during their brief hour of escape from their hothouse and dying like flies with the curious looking at them." Martin's letter followed:

> *Dear Sir,*
>
> *The crime of the decade is being committed here at this World's fair. Under the guise of science and in the name of humanity more than a score of innocent, helpless little human beings have already been done to death, and the dread work still goes on. Protest has been of no avail. Men of prominence fear to take action for fear of scandal, that it may hurt the exposition, etc. What I tell you can be verified by prominent physicians of New York and Chicago who have investigated the matter. The accounts recently published in several of the New York papers do not even begin to do justice to the horrible conditions existing.*
>
> *This "concession," for political and other reasons, was put in the hands of people who did not know the difference between an incubator and a peanut roaster. I see now but two ways to bring this affair to the light of day and have justice meted out and responsibility placed where it belongs—one is*

an appeal to the United States commissioner to the World's fair; the other is publicity and a demand for an unbiased investigation and immediate closing of the place by the Hearst papers.

The first would be a slow process, and in the meantime other innocents would be sacrificed. The second will have an immediate effect and accomplish its work over night.

The first demonstration of the "infant incubator" was made at the Berlin exposition in 1896, since which time it has been demonstrated at all of the great international expositions.

Now, here is the point that makes this "the crime of the decade": Thousands of columns have been published by the press of this country in commendation of the infant incubator. Therefore, to place this affair in the hands of ignorant people, not one of whom has any technical knowledge or experience in this line of work, is to deceive the mothers of this country, whom they send back with nothing but corpses.

Do they have any healthy graduates? When Dr. Hartung made his protest it threw them into confusion. They did not want to increase their mortality rate. A little more than two weeks ago they sent home a child that they had had for many weeks, who, from the treatment received, could not last much longer. Here's what Sister Vincent of St. Anne's Hospital, said:

"The child came back in terrible condition on Friday, and died on Sunday."

The exposition officials would tell you that they have recently made changes both as to the place and the people in charge, and that everything is now all right. A St. Louis dispatch published recently in one of the New York papers said that a secret conference was held, in which half a dozen representative physicians participated. "It was said afterward that it had been agreed that the management of the Pike attraction was doing the best it could, and, with the changes suggested, it was the opinion of the conference that the incubators would do fairly well." The dispatch added: "Several children have died in the incubators lately."

This is incriminating in itself, as it shows that things were wrong. Now that they say it is "all right," I want to ask you: Is the World's fair a place for an experimental station where human life is at stake?

Very truly yours,
Dr. M. A. Couney

Two things are notable about Martin Couney's letter. First, he didn't make any claim to having shown the machines in Berlin. Second, regarding St. Louis, he was right. True, he was a showman who'd lost out to the competition. True, he was dramatic. But he was also in a position to understand that the babies in St. Louis were dying from egregious negligence. While others were hoping to keep this unsavory piece of business politely discreet, he was more than willing to cause a ruckus.

Despite Martin's outrage and the Humane Society's threats, the concession wasn't closed. Dr. John Zahorsky had stepped into the "Charnel House" shortly before Martin wrote his letter. Eager not only to save the day but also to win the admiration of the East Coast medical elite, Zahorsky slowed the march of death, pouring ice water into the coils of the machines when they overheated, sterilizing equipment, feeding the infants breast milk as often as he could, and calibrating feedings. He carefully recorded the weight, the protocol, and the outcome for each infant in his care. When the fair closed on November 30, with the concessions committee's coffers full, he published a series of articles in the *St. Louis Courier of Medicine*. These were compiled into a book—published, to his disappointment, locally by the *Courier of Medicine*, instead of by a major national house.

Zahorksy's words reflect the work of a principled man of science, one well aware of Pierre Budin's recent teachings stressing cleanliness and breast milk. He also cited Harvard's Thomas Rotch, who, despite the failed machine of 1893, remained a powerful force, especially if one had institutional ambitions. (Rotch, unlike Budin, believed "modified" cow's milk was fine; Zahorsky disagreed and had five wet nurses on-site.)

A late-season addition of a glass partition went up between the public and the incubators, on the recommendation of the board of health. Previously, Zahorsky wrote, the babies were subjected to "obnoxious effluvia from thousands of sight-seers." Plus, "the nurses were constantly annoyed by questions." (Martin Couney had no such wall, and questions were encouraged.)

Using graphs and charts, Zahorsky offered detailed recommendations for optimal caloric intake based on weight. Yet he found nasal feeding unmanageable, occasionally mixed "modified" cow's milk (including whey) with breast milk when he faced a shortage, and enumerated numerous blow-by-blow cases of infants dying of vomiting and diarrhea. It's hard to read his accounts and not wonder whether Louise and Maye could have saved more of these children.

Perhaps from a sense of professional courtesy, perhaps from the prudence of ambition, John Zahorsky chose to defend his predecessor on the Pike. Despite acknowledging the overheating machines, "some blunder in the milk supply" and "certain proprietary foods," which he himself discontinued, he still gave Hardy a pass; in fact, he did him the favor of not printing his name. Instead, he picked an easy target, employing a you-know-who-I'm-talking-about plural: "Certain 'specialists' in incubator exhibitions, probably chagrined by the fact that they had not obtained the concession, although they had experience in many other expositions, began to assail the management in every conceivable way." In contrast to the figures stated by the Humane Society, he claimed the mortality rate up to September 1 was only about half. "Consequently," he wrote, "these scandalous vituperations were uncalled for."

The greater damage lay in his assessment of the treatment itself.

Zahorsky hedged his bets. "The feeling of the medical profession is against the show of incubators, of this there can be no doubt," he wrote. "On the one hand there is a prejudice that showmen can not have the proper sentiment toward these little ones and may sacrifice proper requirements of care for show purposes; on the other hand, we feel it degrading to human sentiment to make an exhibition of human misfortunes, especially in the shape of tiny infants." Then he countered with some positives: The show provided free care to indigent patients, it educated the public that "effort should be made to save premature infants and not allow them to die as a matter of course," and careful record keeping would add to scientific knowledge. Fair enough.

But in the end, he blamed the St. Louis debacle on "the catastrophe of hospitalism"—the spreading of germs in an institutional setting—rather than malpractice. ("It was hospitalism that made the mortality so high before I took charge, and it was operative for some time even after radical changes were made in the management.") He concluded that unless a baby's parents were indigent with no other options, the child shouldn't be in an incubation institute—not on the midway and not in a hospital, either. Tiny preemies were better off, he said, at home.

Fear of hospitalism combined with the horrifying specter of St. Louis helped scare the medical profession off the use of incubators. It gave doctors another reason to dismiss a labor-intensive technology they'd been finding hard to maintain. Their disinclination would linger long after the decade in which the crime was committed.

LITTLE MISS COUNEY ARRIVES

New York City, 1907

O n a sweat-drenched bed in upper Manhattan, a woman was writhing in labor. This child was six weeks early. In the frigid dead of winter, the woman's swelling belly would not have been visible under her heavy dresses, her woolen overcoat.

Martin, at the threshold of the bedroom, must have been calculating quickly. He picked up the phone and placed a call.

A final push and the baby was out.

One of Martin's friends, a man with a 90-horsepower automobile, was on his way to Coney Island, an hour each way, to retrieve an incubator out of winter storage.

Meanwhile, Martin plunged the tiny girl into ice-cold water to shock her into breathing.

Both youngster and mother were doing just fine, he told *The Brooklyn Eagle* the following day, along with this mildly improbable version of the entire story. The paper reported that the three-pound newborn promised "to develop into a healthy Miss Couney."

Four adults were living in the Couneys' Harlem apartment: Martin, Maye, her mother, and Louise. Martin was Jewish. Maye was Protestant. Hildegarde Couney was baptized Catholic, as thirty-five-year-old "Aunt Louise," the woman who would raise her, had been. Thirty-one-year-old Maye would have no other children. And no one would file a birth certificate for Hildegarde until 1926.

"WHAT TOOK YOU SO LONG?"

I was riding the train to Brooklyn again, in spite of myself, convinced this would be yet another wasted day.

By the time I arrived at the Kings County probate archive, it was three p.m. "We're closed," the man behind the counter said. Then he relented. "As long as you're here, I guess you can take a look."

He led me to an enormous wooden card catalogue, the kind every library used to have. I figured this wouldn't take long.

Tens of thousands of people have wills on file here. Martin Arthur Couney isn't one of them. *Of course not,* I thought. Then I noticed something: Annabelle Maye Couney had left a will. And so had Hildegarde.

And so I came back and stayed for hours. Louise Recht had a will on file, too, and so did Isador Schulz, the cousin who lived with them in later years, serving as "Dr. Schulz" at Coney Island when the family was away. The wills, for the most part, told the story of money and objects, as wills are meant to do.

Annabelle Maye Couney was the one who had purchased the crypt in Cypress Hills. It had cost her $1,350. An itemized list of assets included a diamond bracelet and a diamond watch and diamond rings and a diamond brooch; and the family's house in Sea Gate, Brooklyn, which was in her name. The inventory listed every silver-plated tray, every platter and bowl and candlestick, every spoon and shaker, sugar bowl and creamer, every glass (one hundred twenty-six, not counting the wineglasses), the bonbon dish and napkin rings (six)—all the stuff of our lives that tells our stories in the language of *things*. This was a tale of company-for-dinner and evenings on the town, of loveliness that sparkled and shone in a beautiful home by the ocean. If only we could reassemble the woman from the jewels, the home from the silver and crystal.

The sole odd thing in this will, and the reason it ended up going through probate, was the special fund set aside for Hildegarde, into which both Isador Schulz and Louise Recht had been putting money. It seemed slightly strange for the nurse to be funding the daughter of her wealthy employers, but who knew?

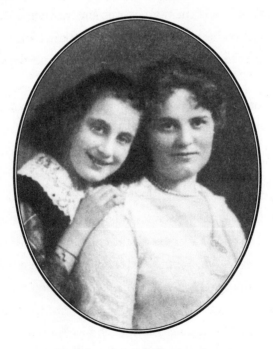

Hildegarde and Annabelle Maye Couney.

Hildegarde's will told a far sadder story. When she died, she was destitute. Her probate folder contained the usual pages of legalese, but where she was buried remained a mystery. In the back of the folder, beneath all the duplicates and triplicates, was a three-page typewritten statement. Anne J. Boylan identified herself as a longtime family friend. "Deponent during the lifetime of Dr. Martin A. Couney, Mrs. Couney and Hildegarde Couney, the deceased, had many conversations with the aforementioned ones concerning the family background, their relatives and their parents and the three of them gave me the following information . . ."

By now I was squirming in my metal chair at my table in the windowless archive, wishing I could jump up and down without looking utterly nuts. Anne J. Boylan's sworn account was riddled with misspellings, including misspellings of names. Some of the information in her account would turn out to be wrong. Perhaps she had misheard or misremembered or perhaps she had been told the wrong thing in the first place. Maybe the person taking her oral statement was tired or bored and dreaming of a day at the beach. Alfons Coney, for instance, was listed as Alfons Torny. Mrs. Couney had no siblings, the statement said, and that wasn't true either. Martin, who'd "invented" the incubators, never held any kind of patent. But what was in these pages was a start—a *real* start.

I tried to imagine Anne J. Boylan in a neatly pressed dress and respectable heels on a hot summer day, setting the record down. Had Hildegarde asked her friend to do this, knowing her days were ending? Had Anne J. Boylan taken the task upon herself? Her words had been waiting sixty years for somebody to find them, long after her own death. As she made her deposition, did she wonder for a moment, *Who will remember me?*

In addition to her testimony, Anne J. Boylan had added another slip of paper to the file. This was a legal certificate of name change from 1903.

Yes, yes, yes, I thought. *Gotcha, Michael Cohn.*

And then I imagined Anne J. Boylan saying, *Well, what took you so long?*

ALL THE PRETTY PREEMIES

New York City and Chicago, 1909

T he headline read, "Wipe Hall with Doctor's Body." Not what Martin wanted to see when he picked up the evening paper, given that he was the doctor in question. And if the words were biliously familiar, it was because he had the original poison pen letter in his possession. He'd have preferred not to share it with the city's bottom-feeding readers.

Maye's cousin Carolina Mastanka had been staying with the family, which had moved to a larger apartment at Hancock Court in Harlem. In slushy February, a scoundrel encountered Carolina at a dance and, claiming he'd fallen in love at first sight, appeared to have taken scandalous liberties.

Martin delivered an ultimatum.

The culprit struck back in arsenic ink.

Dr. Couney:

It has come to my knowledge that you have issued certain statements to the effect that it is impossible for Miss Carolina Mastanka to return to her cousin's home unless she marries me. As your reputation as a dirty liar, far and near, is well known, it is useless for me to deny it. But I write you this to warn you that if you ever again mention her or my name in anything but a respectful way, I should consider it my duty to call and wipe up the hall of Hancock Court with your worthless carcass.

Although I prefer to show clemency to those socially and mentally below me, there is a limit to what I will take. If you are any kind of gentleman and not the coward I consider you, and desire satisfaction, I am willing to oblige you anywhere, at any time, in any way.

> *Very truly, Capt. Paul Mason, late of Nassau Volunteers, U.S.A., and Peruvian Army*

Where, oh where, was Alfons when you needed him? His brother might have scared the cocky britches off the captain by calling his bluff. In fact, he might have roughed him up. Martin, choosing the higher road, hauled Paul Mason before a judge. The latter was ordered to stay away from Hancock Court and put away his pen.

Martin didn't need this kind of attention. Not all publicity was good, despite what Thompson and Dundy might have argued. This scurrilous nonsense interfered with getting people to take him seriously—a pursuit already hobbled by his carnival surroundings.

Maye and Louise could almost always save the babies in their immediate care. To win the larger battle of persuasion, he needed the public's ear. If ever he lost the goodwill of the press, his mission would be sunk.

Often, the Couneys spent at least the better part of the summer in Chicago, where Maye had done her training, leaving Coney Island in Louise's redoubtable hands. A physician named Solomon Fischel worked alongside her. Solomon Fischel was wealthy, and he, like Samuel Schenkein, owned shares in what was now the Infant Incubator Company, a privilege

Martin presumably couldn't afford. Solomon's specialty in Europe had been vision, but the salient issue, as far as the board of health was concerned, was that he was licensed to practice medicine in New York. He could examine a child (if less perspicaciously than Louise), and he could put his signature on a death certificate, an act forbidden to Martin.

The Couneys set up shop in Riverview, an amusement park that tickled Chicago's psyche, as Coney Island did New York's, with a second show in a rival park named White City, after the world's fair.

Chicago's papers loved Couney, the *Tribune* in particular. On June 5, 1905, a coy item peeped out from under the headline "Incubators Save Babies Life" [*sic*]. A child weighing under two pounds had been rushed by private automobile to the White City, and while her identity was held in "strictest secrecy," the paper could divulge that the baby was "heiress to considerable property." Eventually, the daughter of the *Trib*'s own editor, James Keeley, would be rushed to an incubator and saved. But long before that happened, the *Tribune* began hosting benefit days at both amusement parks, with proceeds from the concessions going toward helping the city's newborns. For the 1907 fete, Martin and Maye staged a toddler parade with their graduates dressed up as French dolls. Too cute to resist. And while he was at it, he gave the *Tribune*'s charity 50 percent of the gate.

Chicago was arguably the cradle of American neonatology. Dr. Joseph Bolivar DeLee had founded the city's Lying-in Hospital in 1895 "to succor poor women during confinement." By 1899, the year after the eminent Dr. Martin Counéy made his debut in Omaha, DeLee had two Lion-type incubators; by 1902, he had four. But he struggled constantly for funding, relying on women's charities to keep the obstetrics ward afloat. The primary goal was to prevent mothers from dying in childbirth. He would end up turning his incubators over to a colleague, Dr. Isaac Abt, who founded Sarah Morris Children's Hospital in 1913. Isaac Abt did what he could—which, given his very limited resources, was nowhere near enough.

If you had to be born premature, you'd better do it during the summer, when the sideshows were running. Born in winter, whether in Chicago or New York, you were most likely out of luck.

Not that Martin and Maye were doing nothing. The colder months were devoted to logistics and arrangements for the upcoming season, including hiring doctors—often young ones—to satisfy the local board of health at outposts like the Wonderland Amusement Park in Minneapolis and Revere Beach, Massachusetts. These "assistants" could examine patients, and with the help of the nurses Maye or Louise had trained, they could run the concessions when the Couneys weren't on-site. Once in a while, they had to sign a death certificate. But mostly, this was a sweet gig for a novice doctor, a specialized education wrapped in cotton candy. Just leave it off the résumé. A summer's adventure, and if these young doctors had questions about their convivial boss, they tended not to press. He never made it entirely clear why they, and not he, were filling out paperwork. Sometimes he said that despite his extensive training in Europe, he didn't quite have an American license; other times, he was sublimely oblique.

D r. Julius Hess began his medical practice in Chicago in 1902—the year during which, back East, Dr. Matthew D. Mann and his colleagues continued to bicker bitterly over who was to blame for McKinley's death, and Messrs. Schenkein and Coney were trying to resurrect their business.

Austere, with a commanding presence, Julius Hess was everything Martin Couney was not. After earning a medical degree from Northwestern University, he'd continued his education with postdoctoral work at Johns Hopkins, followed by studies in Germany and Austria. The two men's affects were as different as their training (or lack thereof). Where Martin was effusive, Julius was measured. Where Martin depended on continental elegance to mask a whiff of impropriety, Julius was an incontrovertibly dignified presence. Where Martin encouraged people to call him "Uncle Martin," no one who was not, biologically, Julius Hess's niece or nephew would ever address him as Uncle, nor—a student later wrote— would anyone call him Doc. And only his closest friends would address him as Julius instead of Dr. Hess.

Upon his return to Chicago from Europe, he opened a general practice, and arrived in his horse-drawn carriage at his patients' homes. If, over breakfast with his wife, Clara, a couple of years later, he happened to pick up a paper—say, the *Tribune*, or another of his choice—he would have seen news of the doctor who'd come to town with his baby-saving devices.

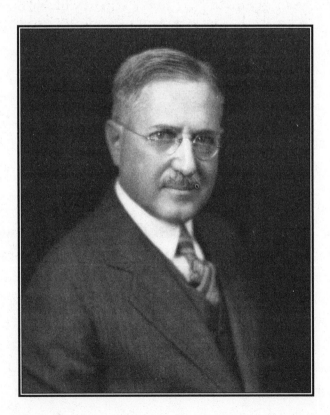

Despite his stiff demeanor, Julius Hess was a man with an open mind. And for all he enjoyed club memberships and accolades, a fine house, a wife—for him, that would never be enough. He was reaching for significance.

In later years, Julius Hess was unwavering and public in his support of Martin. Other doctors would state that it was largely Martin who taught him how to treat preemies, and that he would continue to adapt the showman's ideas. Yet the Chicago physician never recorded precisely when they met. Morris Fishbein would eventually write an obituary for Hess, in which he said the friendship began with Hess serving as the licensed physician when the White City opened. Some of the Couney buffs took this to mean 1914, owing to confusion over when the White City shows ran. The last record of Martin in Chicago's theme parks is 1909, and it's reasonable to suspect the meeting came closer to 1905, toward the beginning of Hess's career.

Julius Hess was six years Martin's junior. For all his reserve and despite their opposing styles, he genuinely liked the showman. Impossible to ignore was the fact that the incubators and the entire system of nursing worked. Although neither man knew at the time, the synergy between their abilities and temperaments would have a profound effect.

More than five hundred babies had passed through Chicago's incubators by the time the 1909 competition for best preemie was held. That Sunday morning, the children were brought to the White City concession dressed in their finest attire. Ruffles and ribbons, buttons and bows. Martin, fluent in baby talk as any other tongue, was having the time of his life.

When the judges selected three-year-old Burton Douglas Stevens of Perry Avenue as the healthiest, handsomest, and best-developed preemie, Martin presented the child with a little red wagon. As had become his habit, he made sure the reporters saw Little Miss Couney, now a chubby two-year-old, with a bow on top of her head.

He also seized the opportunity to state his desire to open a permanent incubator station in Chicago, with government help. He hoped it would happen within a year, two at most. How could it not?

MAGNETIC TAPE

Shortly after Beth Allen suggested that I find Dr. Lawrence Gartner, I realized he had been William Silverman's colleague—the last of the original Couney buffs still living. I also knew that Dr. Gartner was a highly regarded neonatologist, with credentials from Johns Hopkins, Albert Einstein College of Medicine, and the University of Chicago, where he'd been professor and chairman of the Department of Pediatrics and director of Wyler Children's Hospital. He was now professor emeritus of pediatrics and obstetrics and gynecology at the University of Chicago. And he'd been chairman of the board of the American Pediatric Society. I hoped he'd help me—and I figured that before I asked, I should do him the courtesy of knowing what I was talking about, maybe having some information to share.

Armed with Anne J. Boylan's testimony, I was ready. I found an address for a Lawrence Gartner outside San Diego and wrote to him. Three days later, my phone rang. Larry, as he identified himself, remained fascinated by the incubator doctor.

"His name was Cohn," he said.

Oh.

Larry had gleaned that fact from Martin Couney's niece and her

119

husband more than thirty years earlier. But the couple didn't have all the answers. "Was he born in Alsace?" he asked.

"Krotoschin." I had found this on multiple legal documents, including his immigration record, marriage license, and passport application. (A family member would later confirm it.)

"Krotoschin? Where is that?"

And then we were off and running. Lawrence Gartner had cassettes of his interviews with people who'd known Martin Couney during his lifetime. These were made in the 1970s. By the time I came late to this party, the sole living person I'd found who (a) had some connection to Martin Couney and (b) had not drawn breath in one of his machines was George C. Tilyou III, grandson of the founder of Steeplechase Park. Mr. Tilyou was eighty-nine years old when we had a chat. His memory was elusive—I was asking him to retrieve a gleaming sliver from his adolescence. George Tilyou recalled two things. "He was very altruistic," he said. "And he was grouchy."

Grouchy? This was at odds with his public persona. But by the late 1930s, Martin Couney had plenty of reasons not to be in a swell mood. And, as Tilyou noted, one year before his own death, at the age of ninety, it's natural for a teenage boy to perceive an old man as grouchy.

For months, I had been wishing that I could find someone who knew Martin Couney in his prime.

Lawrence Gartner had never transcribed the tapes. They'd been meant for a book he had planned to write, many years ago.

At the end of our conversation, he said, "I am not going to write this book. If you come out to California, I will share the tapes with you."

A DREAM IN FLAMES

Coney Island, 1911

If you want to see something lost rise up again, you can go to the Coney Island Museum and view an exquisite reproduction of Thompson and Dundy's Luna Park, made with 3-D printing. It's the passion project of an artist named Fred Kahl—aka The Great Fredini—who spent more than ten thousand hours creating the 1:13 scale model. You might gaze on its lacy minarets, its balconies and towers, its perfect plastic people, and long to shrink yourself into a past where you've never been.

The love of imagined places fuels extraordinary creativity. We spend our days searching or feeling nostalgia for streets we've never walked, for sights seen only in photographs, for lives we've never lived. The Germans call it *Sehnsucht*. We'll never find what we're looking for, but the pursuit of it has us traversing the globe, or peering into a microscope, or scaling a height, or layering paint on canvas, or stumbling after a ghost.

The last time anyone saw Dreamland standing was Friday, May 26, 1911. William Reynolds, its owner, was determined to finally make his money pit of a theme park succeed. Dreamland ought to be bringing in a fortune, he thought—it was bigger and brighter than Steeplechase or Luna Park—but year after year it confounded him with lousy returns.

Reynolds didn't apprehend that success wasn't simply a matter of concessions. It was the way you played the public. As George C. Tilyou's nephew Edo McCullough would write in *Good Old Coney Island*, "At Steeplechase, if the fact that the mayor was coming on a visit failed to catch attention, somehow the word would leak out that there was a plot to assassinate him in the park, and business would zoom." Likewise, Frederic Thompson would turn the decision to dispose of an elephant into a culture-searing spectacle. "But should Dreamland boast that a local eccentric had invented a new kind of airplane and that a local character had been prevailed upon to fly it from the park to Far Rockaway, it would invariably turn out that the plane would ingloriously pump straight into the drink, and the crowd would shrug its shoulders and disperse, probably to Luna."

Reynolds persisted. For the 1911 season, he'd ditched the all-white theme, repainting the buildings cream and fire-engine red. Eighty-odd lions, leopards, hyenas, and other wild beasts were on-site. Samuel Gumpertz, the manager of the Lilliputian Village, was promoted and put in charge of running the whole operation. Gumpertz was notorious for bringing Igorrote "savages"—indigenous Filipinos first displayed at the St. Louis World's Fair—to Coney Island for a season, an enterprise that got out of control when the tribespeople wanted to leave (and finally went on the lam). If nothing else, Gumpertz had a talent for stirring up drama.

Memorial Day weekend was make-or-break for every showman hoping to survive at Coney Island. Two months earlier, the Triangle Shirtwaist Factory fire left 146 workers dead, most of them young women. New Yorkers needed a reprieve from grief. On Friday, May 26, with the forecast predicting ideal, breezy weather for Saturday morning's season opening, George Tilyou, Frederic Thompson, and Samuel Gumpertz each hoped to get a decent night's sleep. (Thompson's partner, Elmer Dundy, had died in 1907.)

Late that night, a handful of people were awake at Dreamland. At the infant incubator concession, Solomon Fischel had just received a baby from a hospital. This brought the number of patients to five; it would grow as the season went on. Next door was a ride called Hell Gate, which took ticket holders in boats through a dimly lit cavern. It leaked, and workers were putting in overtime to fix it.

By 1:30 a.m., Dr. Fischel had gone to bed. Louise Recht must have been dreaming somewhere other than Dreamland that evening. Instead, a head nurse identified only as Miss Graf was on duty. All was quiet at Coney Island, with only the creatures of the sea scurrying on the beach and the bleary men at Hell Gate toiling thanklessly away. Then an exhausted worker knocked over a bucket of tar. Boiling hot. In a minute, the work lights sizzled and shorted, and Hell Gate burst into flames.

Dreamland was a disaster waiting to happen, with its million electric bulbs and its surface elegance masking shoddy construction (a situation permitted thanks to well-oiled political connections). The breeze that had promised to make for a beautiful opening day carried the flames with astonishing speed. And the water pressure was weak.* With the streams from the firemen's hoses falling short, the inferno was heading straight for the infant incubators.

As the sky turned red and alarms rang out, *The New York Times* stopped the press. In the morning, it would report that all the babies had died.

They hadn't. The best, most detailed description of what happened that night comes from Edo McCullough. As he recorded it, Miss Graf had been just about to wake the two wet nurses for the two a.m. feeding when Solomon Fischel ran into the nursery in his nightshirt. A police sergeant followed. Smoke poured in through the doorway as the doctor grabbed

*Although it was never proven, rumors flew that nearby business owners had illegally siphoned water to protect their assets.

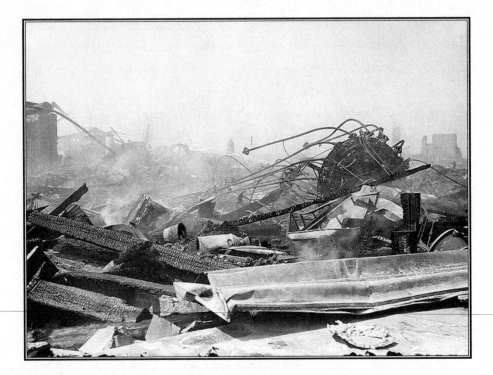

two babies, covering their heads with blankets to shield them. The nurses, still in nightgowns, each scooped up a child; a wet nurse named Anna Duboid grabbed her own newborn, and into the hellish night they fled.

In the utter chaos, the *Times*, along with everyone else, believed the babies had no chance. Ah, but this was always the story with these children. The initial grisly report stated that three had been carried out but suffocated, while "at least three other infants" were trapped inside. The next day's paper ran a correction under the headline "All Well with the Babies." Solomon Fischel explained that he and the nurses had rescued their patients and run to the home of a doctor named John Pierce. "He let us in and we put all five babies into one bed. Then the nursing took its regular course, and in five minutes the babies were as well off as if nothing had happened." Later, he said, he took the babies by taxi to a hospital.

Martin Couney wasn't quoted, which suggests he was out of town at one of his outposts; had he been home, he'd have picked up the phone and put a finger in the dial. He would have wanted to manage the damage, which was considerable, despite Solomon Fischel's reassurance.

Property destruction was the least of it. The initial report of fatalities had ignited the wrath of John D. Lindsay, the president of the New York Society for the Prevention of Cruelty to Children. Despite having been quickly apprised that the babies were safe, he'd dashed off an angry letter to the editor, which ran under Dr. Fischel's account. "That the infants who were on exhibition in the Dreamland incubators were not sacrificed to the fire which destroyed that resort is a mere chance," he raged, characterizing the show as "purely mercenary, violating every principle of medical or professional ethics." He stated that the Society had previously investigated the incubators and had attempted, legislatively, to shut them down in 1906. He concluded with the declaration that such work should be conducted only in hospitals.

But the work *wasn't* being done in hospitals. By the late 1800s, lying-in hospitals, such as the one Dr. DeLee started in Chicago, had popped up in cities around the country, largely to care for poor women who couldn't pay for a private doctor or midwife to come to their home. New York had both the Asylum for Lying-In Women and Sloane Hospital, which had just moved to a new, seven-story building. Sloane would eventually morph into the obstetrics and gynecology ward at New York-Presbyterian Hospital. But expectant mothers with any sort of means chose *not* to go to a lying-in hospital. The protocol was harsh. A few years earlier, a nurse trainee had recorded it: On admission, kerosene and ether were applied to the woman's head, and her hair was washed with ammonia, then braided. Her nipples were cleaned with ether and Albolene. Her pubic hair was shaved unless she was a private patient, in which case it was clipped. After giving birth, she had to lie flat for twenty-four hours and couldn't sit up for the first five days. She could consume only milk—no food—until two full days had passed. For a woman who lived in a squalid, overcrowded tenement and whose days were filled with backbreaking physical labor, this may have been helpful. But someone with a comfortable home would give birth in her own bed.

Sloane Hospital had one hundred cribs for newborns, but it wasn't equipped to care for fragile children in need of long-term care. Few hospitals were, which is why institutions such as the Infant Asylum and Babies Hospital were established in New York. The latter opened its doors in 1887. Eventually, it evolved into Morgan Stanley Children's Hospital at New York-Presbyterian, becoming the sister of Sloane; today it is one of the world's leading neonatal care centers. Early on, however, many of these hospitals' patients were foundlings and children whose parents were indigent, and whatever money there was came from philanthropists and charities. At the time of the Dreamland fire, Babies Hospital and similar institutions were rejecting incubators in favor of less effective padded baskets or warm rooms. Fear of "hospitalism," combined with the labor-intensive cleaning of the machines, argued in favor of an open-air setup. Even taking a baby out of an incubator for a diaper change required more effort than simply picking it up from a basket. Hospitals couldn't spare nurses to sit all day and all night with a single child too weak to suckle. What Mr. Lindsay failed to note in his letter was that there wasn't a choice to be made between a sideshow and an ideal situation. The choice, in many cases, was between a sideshow and letting the children die.

After the babies escaped in the arms of Dr. Fischel and his nurses, Dreamland burned to rubble. And the night saw gruesome deaths. When the fire broke out, the animal keepers freed their charges from their cages, leading them into the main oval arena in order to wait out the crisis. An elephant named Little Hip refused to budge. He would move only under orders from his trainer, who'd been summoned. The animals in the oval stayed calm—until all the lights blew out and the flames shot higher

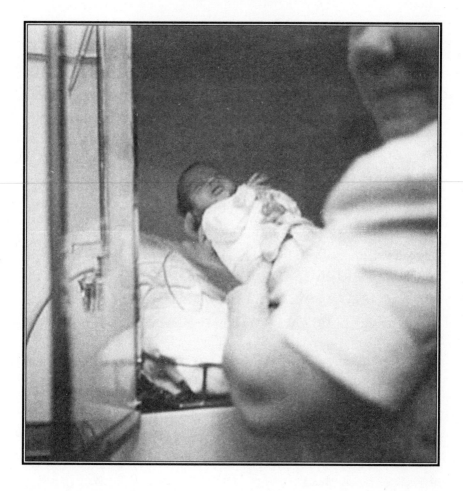

into the night. As it became increasingly obvious that the firemen were fighting a losing battle, the trainers started frantically crating and moving panicked beasts. They managed to get five lionesses and four leopards to safety, and they led the Shetland ponies out of the park by blindfolding them.

Then Dreamland's massive tower collapsed, shooting sparks in every direction. By now the animals were crazed, and any hope of saving them was gone. Some of the trainers stayed and shot as many as they could, sparing them from burning to death. Soon the trainers had to run for their own lives. Little Hip's trainer, who'd raced to the park, had tears streaming down his face as he heard his beloved elephant trumpeting in terror, with no possibility of escape. A three-year-old Nubian lion ran burning through the streets, roaring in agony, with his mane on fire. Police shot twenty-four bullets into the lion's flaming head, finally felling him with an axe.

S olomon Fischel's Saint Bernard was locked for the night in his office on the midway. The doctor had tried to free the dog but was stopped by billowing smoke. Running past flames with his arms full of babies, he shouted to a fireman that his dog was trapped. In a moment of luck and valor, the fireman saved his pet.

But Solomon Fischel's good fortune was coming to an end.

On October 18, 1913, two years after Dreamland burned, he would go to Manhattan's City Hall with a woman named Anna Winter and sign a marriage license. At dinner that night, the forty-three-year-old doctor complained to his friends of feeling ill. Yet the couple went after sunset to a synagogue, where they said their vows in Russian. Next, they checked into a hotel with plans to stay for a couple of weeks. But at four a.m. on his wedding night, Solomon Fischel awoke with a terrible stomachache. Two hours later, he was dead.

The bride fled to her parents' home in Brooklyn as the body lay in rigor mortis.

Louise Recht, learning of Solomon's death, rushed to the hotel. *The New York Times* reported that "physical force had to be used to get her away from the body." She was finally escorted home "in a hysterical condition."

THE FORGOTTEN WOMAN

I had been wanting to pay my respects at Louise Recht's grave, and finally, I got on the train and went. In her will she had stated, "It is my earnest wish and desire to be buried in the family plot of my good friends, Christopher and Belle Egan."

Louise Recht had died with almost nothing and no one. Her only relations were nephews and nieces of predeceased siblings in France. A list of her debts consisted of the bill for her newspaper delivery and her *Saturday Evening Post*. She had set aside twenty-five dollars for Catholic masses.

As I came to the gate at Holy Cross Cemetery, I wished I had thought to bring flowers. Instead, I wandered empty-handed, and despite detailed directions from the woman in the cemetery's office, I got lost. I found the correct row in the correct section, but then I'd count numbers of stones and come up short.

A man in an earthmover finally helped, directing me to a plot I had already passed at least twice. It took me a moment to register that this was the nurse's grave. Whoever Christopher and Belle Egan were, she wasn't buried with them. The marker was for the Hansin family, with five family members' names engraved in the ornate stone. At the very bottom, nearest the ground, was "Amalie Louise Recht."

I stood there a minute, thinking about all the children she'd held and fed and bathed and dressed and sat with through the night, all the wrists she'd slipped through a diamond ring that wasn't hers. Someone had misspelled her name on her grave.

After a while I walked back to the cemetery office. "Just out of curiosity," I asked the woman behind the desk, "is someone named Hildegarde Couney buried here?"

"What year?" she said. And then, "Yes, we have her." She read off the plot number.

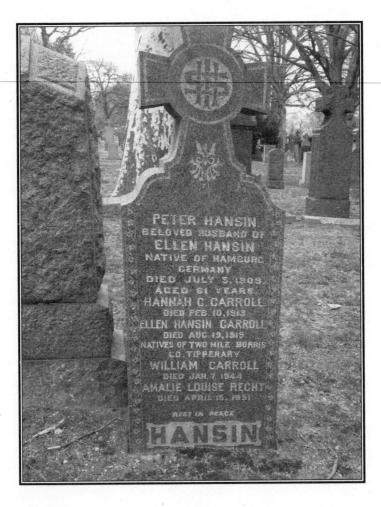

"Is that the same grave I just visited?" I asked. "Amelie Recht?"

She looked again. "Yes, it's the same," she said.

"But there isn't any marker there for Hildegarde. There's nothing at all that says she's there."

"Well, that's where she is," the woman said, before turning back to her paperwork.

BUILDING BETTER BABIES

While Dreamland burned to ashes, a physician named Margaret Clark was cooking up something strange. She had been searching for an answer to a problem: How could Americans breed better children? A generation earlier, Étienne Tarnier claimed to have found inspiration at the zoo. Margaret Clark and her friend Mary Watts found theirs at the state fair. Just as farmers bred heifers and hogs hoping to win a blue ribbon, just as women baked blueberry pies for a prize, mothers might raise better babies for a competition.

Beauty pageants were nothing new, but the women envisioned a different, scientific measure of merit. Points would be awarded for measurable attributes: height, weight, head circumference, and other putative markers of desirable development. Clark and Watts debuted their competition at the 1911 Iowa State Fair—and then the contests spread.

Woman's Home Companion took up the banner, launching a nationwide Better Baby Campaign in March of 1913. The magazine predicted that the initiative would "advance civilization by leaps and bounds" in as few as two generations. If women's organizations and local authorities would kick in the money for sponsorship, the magazine would provide gold, silver, and bronze medals. At state fairs, the highest-scoring city baby and rural baby would each get one hundred dollars in gold. And every baby at every contest would receive a scorecard, pointing out its merits and shortfalls.

Hundreds of pediatricians participated as judges—measuring heads, peering in ears, tabulating scores. Within the first year, forty-five states (out of forty-eight then in the Union) had held a Better Baby competition. Mothers in rural areas and those too poor to pay for a pediatrician were lured by the promise of having their babies examined (at least

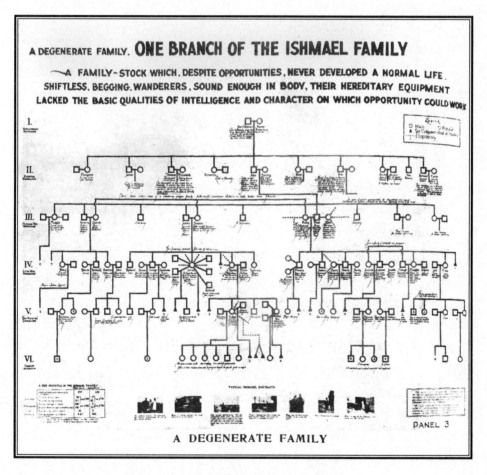

Panel on degenerates from the Century of Progress.

superficially) by a physician, who might make an actual useful suggestion with regard to care or hygiene.

But the downside was appalling. As Alisa Klaus notes in her excellent history *Every Child a Lion*, "The baby health contest was essentially a eugenic concept, and in fact some women's organizations sponsored what they called 'eugenic contests' or 'eugenic exhibitions.'" In time, the score-cards included such criteria as "circumference of chest and abdomen; quality of skin, fat, and muscles; bones of skull, spine, chest, and limbs; shape of eyes and size of forehead; shape and patency of nose; shape and condition of jaw." When it came down to judgment day at the state fair, a "perfect" infant could be only of Caucasian, Western European descent— essentially Aryan.*

True, some of the doctors who judged were focused solely on health and preventing birth defects. (Even Julius Hess himself served as a consulting physician in 1915.) Some had misgivings about their surroundings. But others were bent not only on breeding good seeds but also on ridding the nation of those they deemed bad. A Denver gynecologist named Mary Bates wrote of the contests in terms of her larger goal: to "speed the day when we can have scientific elimination before birth of the unfit, and someday the scientific culture of the fit."

*Once in a while, the organizers held a separate contest for African American babies.

THE DAY OF COUNEY FINALLY ARRIVES

L awrence and Carol Gartner had spent most of their waking hours in hospitals and classrooms in the Bronx and White Plains, New York, in Hyde Park in Chicago, and in Hammond, Indiana. Now they were settled south of San Diego, where snow never fell, and rain seldom did. Their bright, airy house at the end of a winding road was filled with light and colorful artwork. In their early eighties, the Gartners moved with the energy of people far younger. Larry, a slim man with a gray beard and wire-rimmed glasses, had dubbed our meeting "The Day of Couney." Carol, who had retired as a professor of English and the dean of the College of Arts and Sciences at Purdue University Calumet, turned out to be a Couney buff too. She had joined Larry in all his interviews; later, when I listened to the tapes, I would hear her posing some of the less medically oriented questions I'd have asked and think, *Thank you.*

Larry had laid out dozens of folders. I had seen some of the Couney buffs' playful correspondence in the archives of the American Academy of Pediatrics. Now Larry gave me stacks more pages to take back home and copy. "The Couney Newsletter: A Journal Devoted to Making a Great Deal of the Very Little" was one of his own contributions. It was dated May 7, 1970, and marked "Vol. 1, No. 1." Subjects included "Pictures I Have Seen" (including film footage of the incubator doctor shaking hands with a midget), "From the Underground" (Couney gossip currently under investigation), and "Evolutionary Speculations" (Cohen → Coney → Couney).

Larry told me about the German physicians who'd done reconnaissance missions at the behest of the Couney buffs—they had discovered Lion's patent and, further, confirmed that no one named Martin Cohn, Coney, or Couney had ever matriculated in Leipzig; despite two world wars, the city's sole medical school had kept pristine records. A search in Berlin yielded the same result. We talked about Larry and Carol's meeting with Martin Couney's niece and her husband; about my visit to his grave; about Louise Recht's superb care of the babies. The conversation continued back into the kitchen for lunch, and into and out of and through more files. Larry handed me papers in German and fragile cassettes and pages torn out of century-old publications, some with William Silverman's handwriting scrawled in the margins ("Perhaps Couney 'forgot' he had a predecessor"). We talked about the babies. Larry and I both felt there was something wrong with the story of Hildegarde's birth. Who was that child's mother? Carol's mother's friend Gladys—the woman who'd sparked the Gartners' quest—had sworn that Hildegarde was her stolen twin. Both Gladys and her sibling had been in Martin Couney incubators; he told the family the other child died. But the family couldn't accept that. Once, as an adult, Gladys had gotten a glimpse of Hildegarde and saw her spitting image. The problem with this story was that their birth years didn't match—it was a wish to believe in a theft less cruel than death. Eventually, I would come to suspect that Hildegarde's mother was Louise—the physical resemblance is inconclusive—and her father possibly Solomon Fischel, of whom no photos remain. She was devoutly Catholic and he was an Orthodox Jew. In 1906, they would never have married. If something happened by accident during one of their many long summers together, why not give the baby to their childless dear friends? Martin would adore her. "Aunt Louise" would mostly raise her. And Maye would come to like her well enough. Still, Larry told me, there were occasional rumors of hidden dealings, babies—orphans—brokered to would-be parents who wanted to adopt them. Julius Hess and a New York pediatrician named Thurman Givan had investigated once, but found nothing.

The Gartners and I also talked about Alfons and Annabelle Maye, as if these were people with whom we'd become acquainted, and about Martin Couney's more endearing lapses in telling the truth.

"So, Krotoschin," Larry said.

"Well, to be fair, Alfons was born in Alsace—"

"So you think it suited Couney—"

"To be kind of French rather than kind of Polish?"

But beneath the amusement, it was clear that Lawrence Gartner held sincere appreciation. "Did you see that video of Louise Recht feeding a baby?" he asked. He was referring to a film at the pediatric academy archive, and yes, I had watched the dimly lit handheld footage three times. Louise Recht's spoon-to-the-nose maneuver had astounded him and the other Couney buffs: How did that child not aspirate fluid? To me, it had looked like a nifty trick, captured in grainy silence; to someone who understood how hard it was to nourish a child this small, it was a display of skill that elicited a gasp.

I had been smitten with the footage of Madame—sturdy, dark-haired, well into middle age by then—bathing a ribby child so small that its necklace of tiny beads resembles a chain. Her grip is muscular, no-nonsense, as she washes the baby with good old-fashioned soap and water. Squeaky-clean.

From all Larry could gather, the incubator doctor didn't cherry-pick the babies most likely to survive; in fact, he wanted them under three pounds, with some of them under two. Partly, he believed that hospitals could save the four-pounders; partly, he was putting on a show of extreme preemies.

In contrast, Larry told me that when he was a young medical student

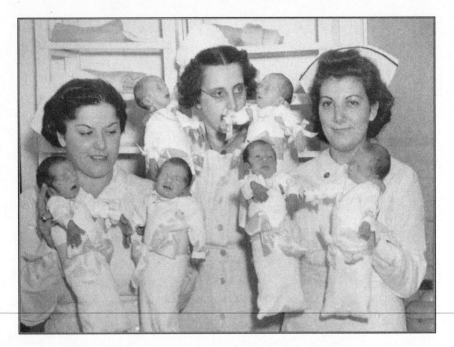

Martin Couney's nurses, with Hildegarde at center.

at Johns Hopkins in the 1950s, if a child was born terribly small, the obstetrician wouldn't even call in a pediatrician. They would lay the baby aside in a warm bin in the delivery room, where it would die. "It was terrible," he said. "And because it was warm they would gasp longer." Perhaps, he said, in what sounded like generosity, the babies had been so small that there would have been no hope. But all these years later, it still ate at him.

On April 29, 1971, Lawrence Gartner had stood in front of a Holiday Inn in Atlantic City. This was the former site of Martin Couney's show, and Dr. Gartner had come to dedicate a bronze plaque on behalf of the Newborn Dinner group. According to the press release, the plaque was to honor "the first person in the United States to offer specialized care for premature infants."

I had seen the undated, handwritten text for a different presentation Dr. Gartner had given, which read, "If Dr. Pierre C. Budin is the world father of neonatology, then Martin A. Couney must be considered the 'American' father of neonatology." In 1970, his fellow Couney buff Dr. L. Joseph Butterfield had captioned a photo of Dr. Couney, identifying him as an "extraordinary progenitor of a new field in the science of medicine" and elsewhere had called the shows "the forerunners of the modern premature nursery." And I had run across written testimony from several pediatricians who were Martin Couney's contemporaries, including Thurman Givan, who said they'd been inspired by him. Givan had organized the Child Health Committee of Kings County in New York, which began to study mortality and morbidity in preemies in Brooklyn hospitals. In light of everything I had heard and read, I couldn't quite grasp the conclusion of William Silverman's original article in *Pediatrics*: "It would be fatuous to attach deep significance to this odd chapter in medical history, especially since the incubator-showman phenomenon was largely the result of the activities of one man." Subsequent academic writings had echoed this sentiment. Why? William Silverman had spent years engaged with his subject, and his article had seemed—to me, at least—to be heading toward the opposite conclusion. Was there something I had misunderstood? Was it simply impossible to credit such an unorthodox, unscientific practitioner in the rigorous world of peer-reviewed publications? Why would the fact that he was alone among showmen have taken away from what he did?

Before the nine-hour Day of Couney ended, at a rib joint down the road, I asked Lawrence Gartner why he thought William Silverman had ultimately dismissed the importance of the incubator doctor. He told me, "I don't know."

The thin spools of tape held the voices of people who'd long ago gone to their graves—their diction, their pauses, their accents, their laughter. The portal to their world. But like that world, Lawrence Gartner's tapes were old. They stalled and snagged, tangled and hissed, and slithered off their spindles. Some were stubbornly blank. A professional restorer said no dice. After multiple tries, I managed to digitize most of them.

One day, a German accent came pouring through my laptop. Ilsa Ephraim was Martin Couney's niece, the daughter of his sister, Rebecca, known as Betty. On the seven minutes of tape that survived, she recalled a tantalizing story about a German exposition in 1898, as her uncle had told it to her. Which didn't make it true.

Ship manifests confirm that Martin *Coney*—new citizen, fresh off Omaha—left New York at the end of that year and returned in 1899, but Ilsa's is the only remaining account of what he was doing there, three years after the famous child hatchery. "There was a big exposition in Berlin, where, after great difficulties, Dr. Couney finally got the permission to show live babies," she said.* In order to make that happen, he'd met with Professor Vincenz Czerny, a gynecological surgeon and professor at Heidelberg, who was a friend of the Cohns. "He told [Czerny] about his plight, that he brought all his stuff along from America and was not permitted to exhibit. And Czerny arranged for an interview with the German empress because he treated the children of the empress's house."

Word arrived that he was to have an audience with the Empress Augusta Victoria the next morning at eleven o'clock in a castle near Potsdam. "Czerny told him how to dress," Ilsa Ephraim said. "He had to wear striped pants, tuxedo cutaway, and high hat and gloves."

According to the story, Dr. Couney hurried to get all the necessary clothing, had the audience, and convinced the empress, who served as the protectress of baby care in Germany. "The show was a tremendous

---

*There is no record of a major exposition in Berlin in 1898 or 1899.

success for him," Ilsa said, despite the fact that "hospitals were only willing to give him the sickest, weakest babies because, when they saw any chance to bring them up themselves, they didn't give them to a showman."

She continued her story: "One year later, his only sister was getting married. They had a very big party for the wedding and as Dr. Couney was still in Europe, he certainly attended this affair and met all the new relatives on his brother-in-law's side. And during the conversation, this exhibit was mentioned. An aunt, very close to the family of his new brother-in-law, said she was there and that a man came, grabbed her, lifted her off her feet and personally threw her out of the exhibit. And Uncle just told her, 'I remember you. And I threw you out myself because you were poking with your finger into the incubators and insisting that these babies were not alive.'

"So it was not a very good introduction to the new part of the family," his niece concluded.

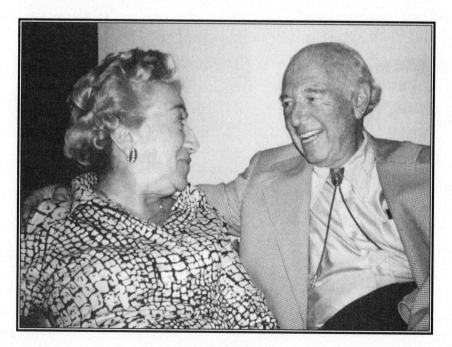

Ilsa and Alfred Ephraim.

I listened again and again, as if repetition would force this belated story to make sense. It has the ring (however thin) of truth; Vincenz Czerny was real. But aside from Betty's wedding, none of the facts add up—nor does the story match any of Martin Couney's well-known tales. It was filtered through time, shaped by retelling and memory, ungraspable yet redolent of the confounding essence of this man.

Breath on glass.

LET'S PRETEND I WASN'T THERE

Denver, 1913

By the summer of 1913, Martin was growing stout. Marriage and fatherhood clearly suited him, and business was robust. With Solomon Fischel manning the East for the final summer of his life, Martin and Maye went west.

Lakeside Amusement Park was the Mile High City's playground. It boasted all the usual frenetic, base-of-the-spine concessions, plus—this once—a show of teeny preemies. His slender young red-haired "assistant"—a newly licensed pediatrician—did such a competent job that Martin had plenty of time to walk the grounds. Back and forth. To and fro. Killing time. Because, sadly, there weren't any medical eminences to wine and dine. After the debacle in St. Louis, physicians turned away. Most of the city's doctors weren't even aware of his show at Lakeside. Those who knew of it viewed it as vulgar quackery, in league with charging admission to see a two-headed calf.

Meanwhile, at the eugenic section of the National Western Stock Show in Denver that summer, on Dr. Mary Bates's turf, the city's esteemed physicians awarded prizes to children with optimal flesh, with perfect ears and toes and noses.

In time, Martin's slender red-haired assistant would become an established pediatrician in Colorado. In the 1960s, Dr. L. Joseph Butterfield tracked him down. The man did not wish to discuss that summer at Lakeside, and given that Dr. Butterfield didn't disclose his name, presumably he asked that it be kept confidential. He found it difficult, he said, "to understand an interest in such a brief event so long ago." When pressed, he conceded that Martin Couney was serious and earnest, and truly desired to demonstrate that preemies could be saved. But the redhead's larger message was, *Don't tar me with that brush.* Whatever knowledge he had absorbed would go uncredited.

KEEP THE INCUBATORS, PLEASE

San Francisco, 1915

Martin had a problem. He had won the concession for the Panama-Pacific International Exposition in San Francisco, but this meant that someone from the Infant Incubator Company was going to have to move west for the better part of a year before the show even opened.

Every conceivable species of minutiae would need to be hammered into submission. Mind-numbing meetings. Memos that flew to and fro in a fever dream of *herewiths* and *we beg to acknowledge receipts*. Ceiling joists and standpipes, water connections, electric work, telephone service, paint colors, gas and contingency gas, suggested protective coating for the temporary building, meter readings, points of egress, fractions of inches between this and that, ad nauseam, ad infinitum.

Solomon Fischel had intended to make his way out to San Francisco as soon as his honeymoon ended. Instead, he died in his wedding bed.* His

---

*A coroner's report would cite "dilation of the heart." Fischel had also suffered from stomachaches for months, but his death remains puzzling.

wife of several hours might have been consoling herself with a hefty inheritance, but Martin was in a fix.

With Solomon gone, Martin would pick up his family and move to San Francisco, but where was he going to find a physician to deal with the board of health? He could always get someone in New York with Louise. But all the way out West? And this was a major world's fair, not a summer stroll in a theme park, where any slender red-headed novice would do. With millions of visitors coming, he wouldn't want Maye to have to train a doctor who'd never touched a baby's bottom. He needed someone suitably impressive. But who?

Julius Hess was mired in aggravation. Yes, his achievements were notable: a pediatric practice in Chicago's Michael Reese Hospital, well on his way to full professorship at the University of Illinois College of Medicine, and soon to be chief of staff at Cook County Community Hospital as well.

He had also invented his own incubator—really, a heated bed. It wasn't pretty like Martin's. It looked like a metal wash bin, a semi-covered bucket on four legs, with a thermometer stuck on top. The view of the baby was lousy; you had to bend over to see it. But Julius wasn't running a show. He was trying to counter objections from his colleagues—that is, among those few who were trying to save preemies at all. The new machine was easier to clean than the incubators Martin used, and its top was open.

Martin's machines were ventilated via a pipeline, through to the outdoors. No matter how nasty and leopard-scented that outside air might be, it was better than regurgitating the nursery's germs into enclosed machines. Infant wards in hospitals, lacking this venting system, were still relying on less effective "warm rooms." Julius Hess was offering the ugly-but-functional best of both worlds: open air, easy care, and individual temperature control.

But no one was taking him up on it.

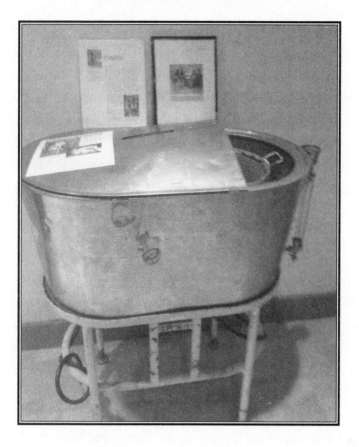

Martin, his improbable co-agitator, believed in the power of public perception. And after Solomon's death, he must have asked Julius for a favor—a large one. Among the records of his many accolades, Julius Hess would save his certificate of participation in the incubator exposition at the San Francisco World's Fair.

All through the spring and summer and fall of 1914, as plans were grindingly drawn and redrawn for the incubator concession, as a shot was fired, killing an archduke and starting a world war, Martin lived on San Francisco's Pierce Street. With him were Maye and Hildegarde, and Maye's ailing mother.

And then there was Alfons, who'd been living in the city for more than a decade. Time had done its work on him. Now in his late forties and childless, Alfons had settled into a salesman's life with his wife, Mary. The Dipsea Race he had accidentally started was now an institution in its tenth year, with teammates who called themselves Indians—complete with chief and grand chief. Destined never to win, Alfons enjoyed his status on the committee and walked the trail two or three times a week. Whether from inattention or from the pleasure of poking in the needle, he persisted in calling his little brother "Dr. Coney."

Frederic Thompson was also in town, and desperate for a comeback. A decade before, with Dundy, he had wowed the crowds not only at Coney Island but also with the mind-bending spectacle of Manhattan's Hippodrome Theatre: elephants and spaceships, clowns and explosions, the id on a bender. Then Dundy died and Thompson drank. And drank. Most of his fortune was gone by the time he lost the last of it in a flammable marriage to an actress. In 1912, bankrupt, he surrendered Luna Park—named for Dundy's sister and not, as everyone thought, for the famous moon ride. Thompson's creditors claimed it. The Panama-Pacific Exposition was his golden chance to redeem himself, with a show called The Grand Toyland. But the magic failed. Thompson fell ill, and never regained his health.

In February of 1915, three days after the fair finally opened for business, a premature baby named Anna was born to parents who rarely caught a break. Anna's mother, Karen Steinicke, had come over from Denmark as a nanny. Her father, Peter Rasmussen, was a stowaway. They met at a Danish dance, and by the time their first child was born—weighing, they thought, barely more than a pound—they were scraping by as a cleaning woman and a carpenter.

What could they possibly do? They put the newborn in a shoebox. And then they rode the streetcar to the fair. The woman who found a place for the baby would have been Maye; the physician who'd save her life was probably Julius Hess; and the man who'd shake the couple's hands and offer reassurance was undoubtedly Martin himself.

Karen Steinicke Rasmussen would ride the streetcar to the concession four times a day, to breast-feed her daughter.

Meanwhile, plans for the fair's Better Baby competition were already under way.

On the opposite coast, Sloane Hospital in Manhattan was gripped by a strange contagion. Nurses and doctors were falling ill, with headaches and weakness, fever and diarrhea. No one understood it. At last, the source was rooted out in the hospital's kitchen. Not the food. The cook. Mary Brown, she called herself. Her real name, Mary Mallon. The health department knew her as Typhoid Mary, a carrier who didn't get sick. Mary had already been ordered never to work in a kitchen. She knew she shouldn't have been there, but the pay was better than working as a laundress. After this infectious misadventure, in which two people died, Mary was arrested. She was quarantined for the rest of her sad life.

Mary Isabella Segner, Maye's mother, was nearing the end. She had lived with Maye and Martin from the time of their marriage. No, she had probably never imagined that her daughter would make a match like this one, to a Jewish showman. Living on the midway, in the midst of clowns and freaks. Yet her son-in-law was good to her. She had been welcome everywhere the couple went. And she loved the child, Hildegarde.

Mary Isabella wrote her last will and testament in San Francisco. In it, she left one hundred dollars to Isabella Russ, her granddaughter by Maye's sister, Frances, who had already died. She left another hundred dollars to Hildegarde. All the rest she bequeathed to Maye, "who has at all times been most kind, loving, and considerate of me," she wrote. Excluded from her will was her other child, Charles, "not, however, out of any lack of love or regard for my said son, but as an evidence of my appreciation to my daughter for her many years of loving kindness to me." Charles A. Segner was a prominent newspaperman in Indiana. Married with children. Given the Segner and Couney families' later apparent estrangement, he might not have taken this turn of events entirely in stride.

While Maye grieved the impending death of her mother, Martin was upset about something else. The fair ended in December of 1915. Rather than tear down a fully equipped facility, Martin wanted to donate it to Associated Charities for the care of the city's preemies. San Franciscans could save these babies if they wanted to; he'd demonstrated how. And yet, at every turn, he faced resistance.

Some of his patients were foundlings or children of the overburdened poor. Sometimes nobody claimed them after the show was over, and they went to orphanages, where no one was going to love them. But did that mean the city ought to simply let them die?

First came the memos insisting that the building be demolished. It sat on private property and the owner wanted it back. But what about the incubators themselves? These were expensive machines. Would no one accept them? Round and round he went with the pencil-dragging bureaucrats.

He couldn't even give the machines away.

The Couneys were still in San Francisco when, on the final day of February 1916, Mary Isabella died. Her will went through probate in Tippecanoe County, Indiana, and was filed in the fall, with Maye pocketing $1,580. Just enough cash to secure a down payment for a property: 3728

Surf Avenue in Sea Gate. Beautiful, exclusive (and quietly, mildly, anti-Semitic) Sea Gate abutted Coney Island, but it was a gated enclave. Captains of industry. Socialites and titans, with white-glove summer homes. In the years to come, the Couneys would live in elegance, along with Aunt Louise. Martin's cousin Isador Schulz would also move in, and never move out.

ONE VERY SHORT LADY

Nedra was seventy-four years old when I found her thanks to Facebook. Her mother-in-law, Anna, was the baby who had arrived at the Panama-Pacific Exposition in a shoebox. Nedra filled me in on the rest: After Anna's parents brought her home, they raised nine more children.

Anna, when she married, took the last name Justice. She bore three living babies, and a stillborn. Her son was Nedra's husband. "She was a very short lady," Nedra Justice said of her mother-in-law, who'd lived to be eighty years old.

Later, I learned that the eugenically perfect winner of the Better Baby competition died of tuberculosis a few months after the fair.

Part Three

THE BLACK STORK

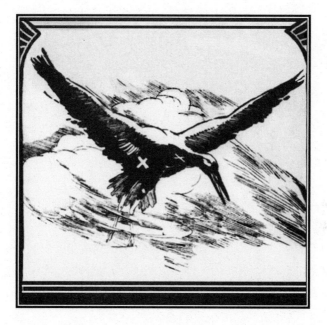

NO-MAN'S-LAND

New York City, 1917

The men had shipped out to fight in the Great War. Some of Martin Couney's earliest patients were among them; one would earn the Croix de Guerre. Julius Hess, though not young, went overseas as a major. In France, Pierre Budin was dead. Alexandre Lion disappeared— his last known show was in the aughts.

That left the littlest citizens in no-man's-land. It wasn't just that the world was focused on the war; the entire approach to birth was in transition. With obstetrics becoming a more sophisticated specialty, middle-class American women were increasingly giving birth in hospitals instead of staying at home. But obstetricians didn't have much time or inclination to fuss over weaklings, and the nascent field of pediatrics hadn't quite gotten to them. They fell between the cracks, where they died.

All the world loves a baby! At Coney Island and in Atlantic City, Martin's patients thrived and so did his business. Women, in particular, kept coming back for a feel-good dose of medical-grade cuteness. One woman would end up visiting the Coney Island concession every week of the summer for thirty-six years.

Slowly, Martin and Maye would acquire the trappings of wealth, in keeping with the neighbors. Crystal goblets on the table, chandeliers casting prisms of light. Sterling-silver chargers under each fine china setting. A servant (live-in) in the kitchen, and a chauffeur (as a matter of safety: Martin did his best, but he was known to be a menace at the wheel). Diamonds for her, black poodles for him. Plenty of room for Little Miss Couney and Aunt Louise and cousin Isador to live in shiny ease.

Martin polished his spiel. He liked to cite the names of famous men who'd entered the world too early:

Sir Isaac Newton
François-Marie Arouet, better known as Voltaire
Jean-Jacques Rousseau
Napoleon Bonaparte
Victor Hugo
Charles Darwin

And who would know the difference if, in spiffing things up, he burnished his credentials? If he said he'd studied in Paris with Pierre Budin, it would strengthen the case he was making to the city's doctors, and cause them to take him more seriously. If he said it was he who'd shown the incubators in Berlin, if he claimed he had European degrees, if he said he'd invented his machines—who was getting hurt? The way the world was, there was nobody checking. Not a soul to contradict him. The truth was, the care the babies got was every bit as good as it would have been if all those credentials were real, and better than any hospital. (One doctor, writing in *The Journal of the American Medical Association* the previous year, announced that "incubators are passé" and "it is a fact that practically all prematures entrusted to institution care die.")

But Martin was starting to paint himself into a corner, albeit a well-appointed one. With the culture changing, he must have felt he needed the credentials—yet anyone believing they were genuine might judge him more harshly. If he had truly been the protégé of Pierre Budin, if he had been educated in Leipzig and Berlin, then it would certainly seem self-serving and exploitative to persist in showing babies on the midway. Why not—at the least—publish clinical results, as John Zahorsky had done? Why not do what Julius Hess was doing, regardless of the frustrations?

Martin Couney had no other recourse. To an extent, like almost anyone of a certain age, he had worn himself into a groove. Too, Maye and Louise had devoted the better part of their lives to this. And money is addictive. But the bottom line was this: He had the means to save thousands of babies, who otherwise were doomed. If he quit, they would die.

What he was offering wasn't only treatment; it was public propaganda on behalf of preemies.

Propaganda mattered in a war. Later, he could have added Sir Winston Churchill to his spiel.

In Chicago, someone else was making propaganda, only his was deadly. Harry J. Haiselden, M.D., was the head of the city's German-American Hospital. Until now, the public had seen two prongs of eugenics. One, at least in theory, was "positive"—it focused mostly on the prevention of birth defects, and prenatal and baby care. The Better Baby contests were an example of this. The second, "negative," prong involved the elimination of "undesirable" births. Before it was over, the horrors of involuntary sterilization would be visited on sixty thousand people in twenty-seven states, including African Americans, Native Americans, Mexicans, people who had committed petty crimes, and individuals with disabilities or mental illness. American eugenics would influence the Nazis, who admired it. Not content to stop at selectively preventing birth, several

American eugenics leaders raised the possibility of killing certain new-borns. Dr. Harry Haiselden unveiled the third prong of the trident. He denied lifesaving treatment to infants he deemed "defective," deliberately watching them die even when they could have lived. In some cases, the traumatized parents were in agreement; in others, he had to persuade them to believe that their children were better off dead. He wasn't the first or only doctor to intentionally allow a child to die, but he was the first to call the press. He eagerly displayed dying babies to journalists, in addition to writing his own articles for the *Chicago American.*

Doctors all over the country lined up on both sides of this fight, as did prominent Americans. Helen Keller, the first blind and deaf person to earn a college degree, famously advocated for the disabled, yet she agreed with Dr. Haiselden. In Chicago, attempts to prosecute him and revoke his license failed. The Chicago Medical Society would finally succeed in strip-ping him of membership, not for letting his patients die but for publiciz-ing his cases.

Meanwhile, frightened parents were writing to Dr. Haiselden, begging him to *do something* about their very disabled children. They had almost nowhere to turn for help, and now they had been convinced their sons and daughters were dragging down the human race.

The movie was called *The Black Stork.* Released in 1917, it starred Dr. Haiselden, coolly playing a character based on himself, in a story loosely based on a real case. In the silent, captioned film, the newborn is afflicted with an unidentified genetic disease. His mother is upset—to be expected—but she accepts the doctor's wisdom after a vision of her child's miserable future on this earth: a life of insanity and crime. When a nurse tries to hand the doctor his operating apron, he sternly refuses her. Chas-tened, she turns and walks away, leaving the infant to die alone on a table. The dead child eventually levitates into the arms of Jesus. One 1917 newspaper advertisement read "Kill Defectives, Save the Nation, and See 'The Black Stork.'"

Later retitled *Are You Fit to Marry?*, the movie played in theaters for years.

The obstetricians sending babies to a sideshow felt uneasy with the spectacle. The parents, too, had their reservations. But what else could they do? In New York, as the years went by, newborns would be coming from Midwood, Zion, Bellevue, Boro Park Maternity Hospital, Long Island College Hospital, Kings County Hospital, and other Brooklyn, Queens, and Manhattan institutions. Over in Jersey, they were arriving from Atlantic City Hospital, as well as the private homes where they'd been born.

Martin Couney's patients didn't have severe anomalies; they were simply early, underdeveloped. But the cultural undercurrent was clear—anyone imperfect, anyone who might grow up with an impairment, wasn't worth saving.

The fire this time began with a cigarette. Midways were notorious for burning, and in August of 1917, a Luna Park ride called the Toboggan, next door to the incubators, burst into flames. This time it was Louise, with another nurse and a couple of cops, who carried all eleven babies to the safety of a hotel.

The incubator show went on: It reopened in Steeplechase Park. And unlike Dreamland, Luna Park survived. Before his career ended, Martin Couney would return. As things played out, the flames of hell might not have sufficed to keep him away.

A CHARMED LIFE

The *New York Times* death notice read: "Appleton—Jean Dubinsky. June 19, 1919–January 3, 2015. A woman of valor, courage and principle. Starting life as one of Dr. Martin A. Couney's famous Coney Island incubator babies, she went on to lead a life of drama and high excitement, participating in some of the most important social and political issues and events of the 20th Century."

I had already spoken with several of Martin Couney's patients, but I had just missed this one. As I read on, I learned that her father, David Dubinsky, was president of the International Ladies' Garment Workers' Union. Among the people she'd met were General George C. Marshall, Bernard Baruch, Pope Pius XII, John Dewey, Diego Rivera and Frida Kahlo, Pablo Casals, Marian Anderson, Orson Welles, Arthur Koestler, Nelson Rockefeller, Golda Meir, Margaret Thatcher, and every U.S. president since Franklin Delano Roosevelt. New York City mayor Fiorello La Guardia had officiated at her first wedding; her second had been to Shelley Appleton, secretary-treasurer of the ILGWU. "Her mind was remarkable to her final days," the obit read.

In other words, I could have called her the week before.

Jean Appleton's daughter, Ryna, who'd written the obit, is a slim, soft-spoken woman. She sat with me at her kitchen table in Manhattan, where she referred to photographs, mementos, and an oral history her mother had done toward the end of her ninety-five and a half years.

Weighing two and three-quarter pounds when she was born in a hospital, Jean was supposed to go to the Coney Island incubators. But an aunt got wind of it, objecting. "My mother's formidable aunt Rose, the proprietress of the famous Dubin's Bakery in Brooklyn, went to the hospital and attempted to grab the baby and take her home," Ryna said. "There was a struggle." Baby Jean wound up in the show, but not before Martin Couney was warned to keep an eye out for Aunt Rose.

I understood my survival was rather miraculous," Jean Appleton told the oral historian. "At a party, I might tell people, 'You never met anyone else who people paid ten cents to see.'"

Her mother took her back for a visit once, when she was about seven. "I remember a very courtly, Old World–looking man and a very cheerful buxom lady," she said.

Ryna had no way of knowing whether that cheerful, buxom person was Louise or Maye, or someone else. But in thinking about her mother, she felt that the incubators had a lasting effect on her personality. "She liked the idea that even at birth, she was something of a 'celebrity.'" She had a will to survive and claim her own destiny.

At the age of five, Jean traveled with her parents to Russia. This was 1924. She saw children sleeping in the streets, and children drunk. A man was dragged and shot—presumably because he had taken a jar of jelly. When someone asked her, "What does your father do?" she replied, "He makes strikes."

"That," Ryna told me, "was my mother's first speech."

Later in life, Jean developed her own passion, apart from her parents'.

She knew plenty of famous designers, but none who'd paid much attention to jewelry—in particular, its cultural and historical significance. She started a program at New York's Fashion Institute of Technology and founded the American Society of Jewelry Historians.

Ryna described her mother as "elegant and vital." She was "well read, a student of history, a Francophile, and interested in the new." In her final years, she used an iPhone, an iPad, a computer, and an e-reader.

What Jean Appleton said in her tenth decade was, "I had a charmed life. It was my Arcadia."

THE RISE AND RISE OF JULIUS HESS

Chicago, 1922

J ulius Hess, back from the war, was embarked on a life-and-death
mission. Hard as it would have been to miss the arrival of Martin
Couney in Chicago way back when, it would have been impossible
not to notice the murderous exertions of Dr. Harry Haiselden. Not every
preemie would grow up unaffected by its birth; some would have physical
or intellectual disabilities. And often enough, prematurity was caused by
syphilis, which carried the stigma of "bad breeding." Someone needed to
defend these children, fast.

Having created his own machines, Julius Hess's next salvo was to write
a book. *Premature and Congenitally Diseased Infants*, published in 1922, contained hundreds of pages of case studies, diagrams, photographs, charts,
graphs, and X-rays, the solid earth beneath Martin Couney's airy verbal
flourishes. Hess made the distinction between "preemie" (born preterm)
and "weakling" (full-term but underweight with difficulty thriving), although the words were tossed about interchangeably in general public discussion. He was fighting for both, and he left no ground uncovered.
Primary causes were cited, which, in addition to syphilis, included poverty,

illness, stress, and multiple births (twins and triplets). Development of critical human organs was interrogated in detail. Diseases, and feeding, and heat, and nursery design were analyzed, along with every conceivable protocol, including what oughtn't to go in the wet nurses' mouths: aromatic vegetables, unripe and acidic fruit, fried meats, rich pastries. (Not a word regarding beer, which a certain young showman had once endorsed.)

Hess's book was the first nationally published American volume in the emerging science of neonatology. It was urgent, he wrote in the preface, because prematurity was on the rise in Chicago, and because, "in the United States the care of premature infants has not received the general attention of the medical profession which it merits." In the final pages, he listed the names of more than one hundred fifty physicians around the world whose work had influenced him, including Budin, Tarnier, and Credé. But he cited just one man in the preface: "I desire to acknowledge my indebtedness to Dr. Martin Couney for his many helpful suggestions in the preparation of the material for this book."

T hat same year, Julius Hess used a donation of $10,000 to open the Premature Infant Station at Sarah Morris Hospital, with an additional $900 a year. Two years later, the Infant Aid Society of Chicago stepped up with what would become an $85,000 endowment, naming the station for the charity's founder, Hortense Schoen Joseph. In the interim, the Society kicked in another $5,000 a year for operating expenses. It wasn't enough. But at least it was a start.

In 1924, he had a dozen Hess beds, and a heat lamp, and a portable ambulance he had designed. And in walked an exceptional nurse named Evelyn Lundeen, who would work with him for the rest of his life.

A LEGEND IS BORN

Coney Island, 1922

Step right up, ladies and gentlemen! Every summer, the barkers showed up at Coney Island, most of them dreaming of acting careers. Stumbling around on stilts, squished between sandwich boards, hoarsely exhorting crowds to see the latest, greatest, unforgettable whatever-the-heck wasn't exactly heaven, but it would have to do until vaudeville or Broadway called.

Martin Couney's barkers took a tone decidedly soberer than their fellows'. No sandwich boards for them. But business was business, and he needed them, these sonorous men who wooed you in: *"Don't forget to see the babies!"* Inside, character actors also served as lecturers. One barker alum, Don Carney, went on to be "Uncle Don," a popular children's radio host. Another was said to have become a diplomat.

The most delicious story involves a British youth named Archibald Leach. In the summer of '22, Archie allegedly stood outside the incubators, beckoning the masses while awaiting stardom. A minute later, Archie was Cary Grant.

The man who really hired him was George C. Tilyou, who handed

Archie a green coat with a red braid, a loud green cap, a pair of stilts, and forty bucks a week—not a bad salary then. But in the 1960s, the movie star looked back on this gig with something less than fondness: "Y'see, with the children out of school roaming around looking for something educational, my tall figure presented a tempting target for aspiring Jack the Giant-killers. . . . I could predict the concerted rush, and spot the deceptive saunter resulting in the rear-guard shove; or the playful ring-around-the-rosy, with me as the rosy, beaming daffy down on the little faces of impending disaster. I dreaded the lone ace who came zeroing in out of the sun, flying a small bamboo cane with a curved handle. One good yank as he whizzed past and he'd won the encounter hands down (*my* hands down), with full honors and an accolade from admiring bystanders."

Archie Leach was out of there fast. Did he ever take a pratfall in front of the incubators? Sub in for a friend on a rainy day? Stop by for a wink and a peek? I asked George Tilyou's grandson George III. He recalled only that "Cary Grant was a stiltwalker. My uncle Edward met him and he said something about going to Hollywood."

As for his incubator stint, it's another beautiful Coney Island tale: If it isn't true, it should've been.

ALONE IN A CROWD

Coney Island, the Roaring Twenties

Y ou would think that Julius Hess's written thanks would change the conversation, and you would be wrong. No matter how Martin embellished his own credentials, no matter what Julius said in his favor, it didn't improve his standing to the extent he'd hoped. People seemed to think the Chicago physician had a quirky affection for the showman, and don't we all have a couple of peccadilloes?

While Julius was setting up his hospital, Martin competed for quarters with the Alligator Boy. He used no medicine other than whiskey (a drop a day per baby), but he had started giving oxygen to the most underdeveloped infants, as did Julius. And he was equally strict about the wet nurses' diets. Later, he'd claim he would fire any wet nurse who noshed on a hot dog (who knew what was in those?) or sipped an orange soda (God forbid). But he was on his own.

If Julius felt discouraged, he nevertheless had colleagues, professional community, a place where he belonged.

Not Martin.

Even if physicians bought his story, even if his tony Sea Gate address impressed them, even if they were happy to dine on his tab, even if they sent him patients and saw the babies thrive, in the end, he would never be one of them.

Then there were the rumors. For years, Samuel Schenkein held shares in the Infant Incubator Company, but finally, he was out. The business was owned solely by the "family"—Martin and Maye, Louise, Isador, and another pair of cousins. The Couneys' increasingly lavish spending—the new construction improving their home, the frequent trips abroad—and even the lines around the concession, all of it made him a target of suspicion. Some critics persisted in thinking the babies weren't real. That was harmless nonsense, but others accused him of baby-swapping or baby-stealing, crimes that could make a man rich. The lack of evidence did nothing to deter them. Just as no one demanded he prove his credentials, no one required his accusers to offer any proof. One journalist asked him point-blank about the "rumors" (never saying what they were) and reported he'd laughed them off. "I'm not surprised to hear there are rumors about the babies," he said, "for the general public is entirely ignorant of what we are trying to do. We don't tell people who the babies are, naturally, and after they leave here they are so changed, no one could possibly recognize them." He swore that the board of health and the hospitals knew his record was clean.

The one public story about an adoption was back in 1916: A woman identified as Mrs. Richard Elkins took home a baby whose father was killed in the trenches in Flanders and whose mother had died after giving birth. Mrs. Elkins gave the child her family name—Lonsdale—rather than that of her son-of-a-senator husband, suggesting some interesting negotiations.

If Martin did anything else, he buried the evidence so deeply that it has never been found. But even supposing he brokered adoptions for profit, the ethics of it are tricky. The alternative for orphans would have been a foundling institution—where mortality rates were high, especially for a child weighing five or so pounds and still needing special care—as opposed to a loving home. Regardless, for the rest of his life, Martin would deny having done it.

Occasionally, he said, a couple who'd been married, say, seven or eight months would try to bribe him to take the baby and say it was premature. He refused.

However, he was open to taking donations from grateful parents. Even those of few means often gave him *something*. And if a rich family whose baby he'd saved *insisted* on giving him money, was it so awful to take?

M artin didn't like taxes any more than he liked death. He'd been filing as a "personal service corporation"—essentially a charity—because, although he charged admission, he didn't bill his patients. Was this not a personal service? The IRS thought not. Eventually, he took his case to the U.S. Board of Tax Appeals. The board ruled against him, requiring him to pay up.

E qually distressing was the Coney Island cop who had it in for him. For forays of more than a couple of miles, Martin relied on his driver. But the locals knew Martin. He was not drunk. His zigs and zags were generally indulged as he drove to his concession.

On July 23, 1926, Patrolman Thomas Toolan directed Martin to turn his car into a Coney Island parking lot, but he wanted to continue on the road. "You go where I tell you to go," Toolan said. And then it got ugly.

In minutes, Martin was arrested and charged with disorderly conduct. He would later say that the patrolman made him drive to the Coney Island Precinct. Once there, Toolan conferred with a lieutenant, and the two came back, accused him of grazing Toolan's leg with his car, and set bail at $500.

Martin called Louise, who went to fetch the cash, but before she could even come back, he was "hurried out of his cell, put into a patrol wagon, and taken to Adams St. Court," in downtown Brooklyn, he said, adding that they'd handled him roughly, hurting his arm. His hearing was set for August 8.

For his day in court, Martin took no chances. His fifty character witnesses included Edward Stratton, publisher of the *Coney Island Times*, and Samuel Gumpertz, former importer of Igorrote tribesmen, past manager of the incinerated Dreamland, and now the respectable president of the Coney Island Board of Trade.

The charge was dropped.

The Coney Island showmen and promoters had his back. They respected Martin for his tenacity and class. But no, he wasn't one of them, either. In a strangest-thing-ever-at-Coney-Island contest, some might have cited the Elephant Hotel, but others wouldn't blink before picking the incubator guy. He was the thing that didn't go with the others.

Peruse *The Brooklyn Eagle* on an average day, and you might learn that Dr. and Mrs. Martin Couney had made a donation to the Democratic League, or that Miss Hildegarde Couney, having attended the College of Mount St. Vincent, was now sailing on the *President Roosevelt* for France. There she would finish her education at the Lycée Victor-Duruy Academy for Young Ladies. You might read that Miss Couney had been awarded the Diploma of Honorable Mention for Languages while in the City of Light.

But within the lovely, cultured company the Couneys kept, Martin failed, yet again, to qualify as *one of them*. He was still a showman. And darling, that name and those airs didn't fool them: He was Jewish.

SEND THE AMBULANCE

Atlantic City, the Great Depression

The stock market crashed. Women's hemlines plunged. The rate of prematurity shot up. Martin blamed this rise on mothers being overworked and stressed and poorly nourished. And he was growing starchy. He disapproved of a pregnant woman snatching a lettuce sandwich on her noon hour and calling that lunch. Nor did he like her going to a motion picture show instead of resting at night. "Things were different a couple of decades ago," he told a reporter. "The women stayed at home and cooked three square meals a day, and exercised, and got plenty of fresh air and good food before the birth of each child." The expectant mother, he added, "wasn't worried about where the next meal would come from, as young mothers are today."

But he couldn't revert to a time that probably never existed (except in his rosy memory) for most urban women. And he certainly couldn't subvert the allure of the motion picture shows. They were as Depression-proof as he was. His Luna Park and Steeplechase neighbors stalked the weekly newsreels. The minute a promising misfit flashed on screen—say, a guy who could toot a horn with his ear—the bidding war began.

171

Martin just kept working. If a mother was broke, he might hire her while her baby was in the show, sending her home in the fall with a healthy child and a livable nest egg. With both the Coney Island and Atlantic City concessions at capacity, Maye worked hard to find spaces for the babies, and Martin went back and forth.

In Atlantic City, admission was by donation, a possible end-run around the IRS. At Coney Island, he was still charging a fee. Once in a while, a parent sniped that he should've gotten a cut of the gate because Martin was getting rich off his kid, but most were deeply thankful.

In 1932, Martin began to notice the frequent visits of a Steeplechase electrician. The young man, who'd once been his two-pound patient, was now a regular presence.

"Such a grateful boy," said Martin to his night nurse.

"Isn't he, though," she answered.

But he was also arriving late at night, hoping Martin wouldn't wake up.

Finally, the nurse and the electrician informed him they had married. "Scoundrels," Martin joyously told a reporter.

But his deepest pride was Hildegarde, working as a nurse in Atlantic City.

Little Miss Couney hadn't sailed happily into adulthood. Rumor was, she had lost someone she loved in the Great War. Also that she'd drunk moonshine during Prohibition, and suffered temporary blindness.

Despite being shipped off to Paris, to a school where young ladies were "finished," Hildegarde Couney would never be dainty or ladylike. People called her "mannish" and "hefty" and "prickly." *Not pretty* went unsaid. All her life, whether she liked it or not, she would serve as a sample preemie, and her girth was news: She weighed 135, she weighed 160!

After Paris, Hildegarde's next stop was the nursing school at Atlantic City Hospital, not far from the incubator station on the boardwalk. She became an R.N., mastered Aunt Louise's spoon-to-the-nose technique and the entire repertoire of baby-saving moves.

Soon enough, she would be at the center of a national drama.

D r. E. Harrison Nickman was Hildegarde's professor and a pediatrician at Atlantic City Hospital. He also worked at the incubator concession. "They were absolutely fabulous with these babies," he told Lawrence Gartner almost forty years later. By the 1930s, few of the "helpers" were novices. "There was this custom to find the top pediatrician in the area and have him take care of these premature charges. Actually, in getting the top pediatrician, to a certain extent, [Martin] was *training* the top pediatrician.

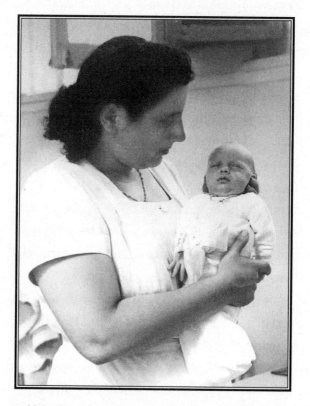

Hildegarde would come to run the Atlantic City concession.

He had innumerable contacts. For example, when the AMA would meet in Atlantic City, this premature station on the boardwalk was a hangout for all of the university professors."

Atlantic City Hospital was among the biggest in South Jersey, yet when it came to preemies, the hospital had no facilities. Instead, someone would send the ambulance driver, Jerome Champion, off to the boardwalk with the newborn and a nurse, or they would send him out to a private home to fetch a patient. Even the family who owned one of the biggest hotels on the beach sent their infant to the concession. No amount of money could've bought anything better. "It's the first time I ever saw oxygen piped into a series of units. He had a pipeline just like we have now," Dr. Nickman said in 1970.

"I've never seen a hospital as clean as that place," he added. "Not only was the nursery clean, the place where the people circulated was clean. Anybody that dropped anything, it was picked up right away. Absolutely immaculate."

Dr. Gartner had a few additional questions before concluding his interview. No, Dr. Nickman never once saw Dr. Martin Couney examine a baby. Nor did he ever see him pick up a medical journal.

The news was like a fly in Martin's ointment—a baby in Kansas and another in Michigan weighed a scant pound, the papers said. An Ohio child tipped the scales at fifteen ounces. Impossible, he countered. For backup, he telegraphed Julius, who concurred.

Then he acquired his own headlining preemie. Born at Long Island College, Baby Arlene weighed between one and a half and two pounds (her doctors didn't even bother to weigh her the day she was born). Martin came and fetched her in a heated basket, and sat in the back of the car while his chauffeur drove them out to Atlantic City.

In May of 1932, he mailed her mother a Mother's Day card and signed it "Arlene." In June, her parents came to retrieve her, thwarting a frequent visitor who begged to adopt the child. Maye dressed her in a woolly pink jacket and a pink bonnet, and wrapped her in a soft yellow robe. "Feed her 2½ ounces of milk seven times a day, steel yourself against her crying if she wakes up in the night, come back to us every two weeks so that we can see how she's getting along, and take good care of her," she told Arlene's mother.

"I think I love her as much as her parents," Martin told a reporter. "I can't understand why some people still think these premature babies aren't worth saving."

A t any one time, he didn't have room for more than fifty newborns, and he was covering all of New York City and Long Island and southern New Jersey. In winter, he didn't have any facilities at all. In Chicago, Julius Hess was forced to turn patients away. The showman and the physician were getting on in years. There had to be *something* they could do to make the entire country pay attention.

And then there was.

THE CENTURY OF PROGRESS

Chicago, 1933

On May 27, 1933, light that had traveled across the universe from the red giant star Arcturus kindled a brilliant Deco city. The starlight had supposedly started its journey in 1893,* the year of the Chicago Columbian Exposition. In an act of magical planning, the minds behind Chicago's second world's fair built the Adler Planetarium, and used it, along with three other planetariums across the country, to capture the star's rays, converting them into electrical power.

Then they threw the switch.

The year 1933 was the bottom of the Depression. Violent storms of dust choked the plains. Gangsters bloodied the cities. Pantries were bare and the news was bleak. On January 30, Adolf Hitler became chancellor of Germany. On February 15, Chicago's mayor, Anton Cermak, was hit by a bullet intended for Franklin Delano Roosevelt. The mayor was standing

*This calculation was probably off by a few years.

next to the president-elect at an event in Miami. Cermak lingered a few weeks, and then he was dead. On February 24, Japan withdrew from the League of Nations. In March, Hitler consolidated power.

Prideful and defiant, Chicago threw a party, and everyone was invited. The minute the switch was thrown, rainbow colors blazed along the lakefront, turning the drizzly night into a vision of hope and promise. By August, more than a million people were paying to visit each week. Today might be glum, but look at what's coming!

The only thing missing was irony. In *Harpers Magazine*, Ludwig Lewisohn took a rare contrarian view, arguing that technological advance was *not* the same as human progress: "Flagrant above all other examples and illustrations of the fallacy that in this machine age we are thinking new thoughts and creating new morals is that delightful machine or group of machines by means of which, sitting in a darkened hall at our ease, we can see far lands strange as dreams which we shall never visit."

But for most everyone else, the fair was a beautiful valentine to the future. And what better valentine to the future than a baby?

The pink-and-blue concession on the midway had a big assist from Julius Hess, and help from Herman Bundesen, the health commissioner. The fair's Executive Committee stepped up, too, and arranged for extra funding through the Infant Aid Society. Chicago's Lying-in Hospital supported the exhibition. Sarah Morris Hospital sent every preemie patient to the midway, along with the reluctant Miss Evelyn Lundeen. Some of the weaker and sicker infants stayed in Hess beds, kept in back, not on display, but they, too, were part of the Century of Progress.

Julius Hess had spent the previous decade producing clinical results. Dedicating a 1928 text on infant feeding, he wrote: "To Dr. Martin Couney, I affectionately inscribe this effort to put into practice the experience of a quarter century. The thoughts on feeding premature infants were largely stimulated by his devotion to the welfare of these small infants."

These two men depended on each other more than ever. Martin needed respectability, while Julius lacked one critical thing: a propaganda machine. Eleven years after Sarah Morris opened its premature ward, he didn't have the money he needed, and he was never going to get it without public opinion on his side. Martin had no charts or graphs, statistical analyses, nor could he publish in medical journals. But he knew how to touch the hearts of ordinary people—the kind who paid taxes, the kind who had babies, the kind who, having come from the fair's well-funded exhibition on eugenics, didn't see why anything ought to be done for the runts.

Sally Rand, performing her sexy fan dance right next door to Martin, would have succeeded without the help of Chicago's police, but getting arrested for indecency was wonderful for business. (Legend has it that she quipped she was wearing more than the babies, so what was all the fuss?) Did she ever stop in to visit the little mites? Did Martin sneak a peek at her? He was a busy man, pumping hands, holding court, feeding doctors, answering questions, calling Atlantic City, where Hildegarde was in charge, and Coney Island, where cousin Isador ("Dr. Schulz") took care of things. For someone who'd spent most of his summers at Sodom by the Sea, Martin was puritanical. Eventually, he requested that a barbed-wire fence go up between concessions so people couldn't jump the gate from his to hers. Still, he was only human.

If ever he walked the fairgrounds, he'd have gotten an eyeful. The eugenics show—the first (and last) at an American world's fair—was just for starters. This particular exhibit was devoted to the eugenicists' second prong (preventing undesirable births). Their Nazi friends across the sea would be the ones to take the third prong—murder—and twist it into its final shape. Leaving the Hall of Science for the midway, Martin could have seen a show called "Life." At its entrance was a picture of a stork with a two-headed human fetus; inside, you could see a dead creature floating in a jar. Nature deleting mistakes. Grotesque as it was, it was less heinous than its sophisticated counterpart, with its patina of scientific endorsement.

On the evening of July 3, Martin might have meandered to Soldier Field for Jewish Day—although he probably didn't. On July 15, he could have viewed the arrival of twenty-four Italian seaplanes led by Italo Balbo in a show of fascist power. Had he been so inclined, he could have strolled to the fair's Indian Village, where Chief Blackhorn adorned Balbo ("Chief Flying Eagle") with a headdress. On October 26, with the fair still going strong, he might have seen the German airship *Graf Zeppelin* circling the lakefront displaying its might—and he probably did; it was the talk of the town.

He might have regarded the stars at the Adler Planetarium or the bones at the Field Museum. He could have perused the Time and Fortune Building, sampled (and dismissed) the mayonnaise at Kraft Food Hall. He could have beheld with awe the Lama Temple or the Hall of Religion, or Travel and Transport, with its roof that "breathed."

It's within the realm of possibility that, stepping outside his concession, as millions of people walked by or went through, he winked, unseen, at a teenage boy whose name was William Silverman.

Barbara Fishbein, whose father, Morris, was the editor of *The Journal of the American Medical Association*, accompanied him to a gourmet dinner at the Couneys' almost nightly. Years later, she'd recall that her host professed to have learned his culinary skills while working as an aide to a general in France during the Great War. (Cue Maye quietly rolling her eyes.

But of course, the army would send a middle-aged Jewish showman to do the gourmet cooking in France. Martin had no military record.)

Before he left Chicago, Martin gave Barbara Fishbein a gift.

Martin Couney's Spaghetti Sauce for Newlyweds

Olive oil

1 clove garlic, minced

1 large onion, diced

1 lb. hamburger

1 can tomatoes

1 can tomato sauce

1 can tomato paste

Salt, pepper, herbs to taste

Cover the bottom of a two-quart pot with olive oil; brown garlic and remove; add onion and hamburger and lightly brown. Add rest of ingredients and simmer one hour.

NOT FOR PUBLIC VIEWING

Memorial Day, 1934. A woman ate a hot dog at a party and regretted it. (Martin would have told her not to do it.) Really, she felt awful. Oh, and she was nine months pregnant with twins. She was rushed to Chicago Lying-in, where as her blood pressure surged, one of Dr. Joseph Bolivar DeLee's associates performed an emergency cesarean section.

The babies, Barbara and Joanie, were full-term but underweight—weaklings in Julius Hess's book. Their mother had toxemia. Size-wise, the twins were a lopsided pair. At four pounds, Joanie could stay in one of the incubators at Lying-in until she put on a pound and was healthy enough to go home. Three-pound Barbara was sick and given little chance to live.

When I spoke with Barbara Gerber, she was eighty years old. She lived in California but had grown up on Chicago's South Side—she recalled skating in front of the University of Chicago, "where they were probably building the atom bomb, but who knew?" And she told me about her birth. She was transferred from Lying-in to Sarah Morris, sick and needing to be transfused. Her father couldn't afford that, she said, so the nurses snuck him in to give his own blood to his daughter.

When all the Sarah Morris patients were sent to the Century of Progress, Barbara was kept in the back with the sickest babies—the ones the public never saw.

Three months passed. "My parents got a call to take me home to die," Barbara said.

"Really?" I was shocked. This was the first I'd heard of Martin Couney calling it quits on anyone, ever. But in reality, he wasn't her physician.

"I guess I didn't improve very much," Barbara said. "My mother's story was that they carried me out, and I took a deep breath and took off running."

Her twin, in contrast, suffered lifelong health problems, including a collapsed lung, and Barbara wondered whether some of them could have been traced to the time she spent in the incubator at Lying-in. Joanie died at the age of forty-eight.

"Is there anyone else from the class of '34?" Barbara wanted to know. Then she wanted to know who else I'd met from *any* year. And she wanted to meet me in person. She would be going to Long Beach, Long Island, in a couple of months. And that's how a plan began to take shape.

ALL ABOARD THE TWENTIETH CENTURY

Chicago, 1934

At Ripley's Odditorium on the midway, a two-year-old named Betty Lou Williams was causing a sensation. One of fifteen children born to impoverished sharecropper parents in rural Georgia, Betty had a beautiful brown face, an extra arm, and a pair of stunted, helpless legs emerging from the left side of her torso.

Rich or poor, in 1934 no surgery could have made Betty resemble other children. Her choices were to live in isolation or make a substantial fortune as a freak. After the fair, she traveled the country and her income shot up to as much as $500 a week. Betty provided for her siblings, putting them through college, before she died at the age of twenty-two.

In the most famous photo of her, Betty is hugging herself. She looks as if she has somebody else alive in her body, craving escape.

The situation in Europe was getting worse. June 30, the Night of the Long Knives, was the start of a violent purge of the Nazis' political enemies; people who thought Hitler wouldn't last long were losing heart.

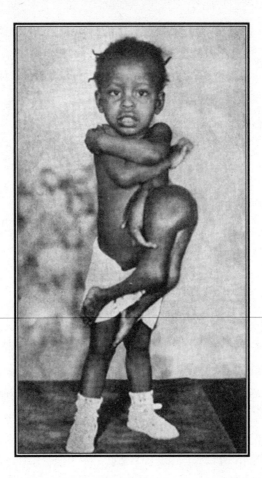

Martin's sister, Betty, had emigrated for Palestine, but his young niece, Ilsa, remained in Berlin, and he feared for her.

Meanwhile, Maye's brother, Charles, lived in town. He had been the managing editor of the *Chicago Evening Post*, but there is no mention or record of his dining at the Couneys' table. Perhaps because he'd lost the inheritance in favor of Maye, or perhaps because his brother-in-law was not his type, he may have kept his distance.

Chicago partied on. This second summer hadn't been in the original plan, but the fair was going to have to run for another season if the backers were to have a prayer of turning a profit. This year's program guide read,

"You have come here to see in epitome the great drama of man's struggle to lift himself in his weakness to the stars."

Sally Rand was back and, having ditched her feathered fans, was dancing in a giant bubble, which resembled—arguably—an amniotic sac.

Halfway through July, Chicago inaugurated a gift from Benito Mussolini. The engraved Roman column was given in thanks for the warm welcome of Italo Balbo and his seaplanes the previous year.

Balbo would die in 1940. Almost every structure from the fair would be dismantled. But the column stands. You can find it in Grant Park.

Ten days after the column's inauguration, the infant incubator reunion, broadcast live, went off without a hiccup. Of the previous summer's seventy patients, twenty-six had died—thirteen within the first critical twenty-four hours. That's quite a bit less than the 85 percent survival rate Martin always touted. But subtracting the babies who didn't last a day (which the great Pierre Budin did as well), you come close. The smallest survivor weighed only one pound, ten ounces at birth, and two others were under the two-pound mark. The achievement was significant, and Julius Hess was keeping careful track.

All but two survivors came to the reunion. Prominent doctors and members of the Infant Aid Society stood by as Herman Bundesen took the microphone. After beginning with "All the world loves a baby," he stole the rest of the showman's spiel, invoking Victor Hugo, Napoleon, Voltaire, Rousseau, Newton, and Darwin. And he pointed out "splendid opportunities" for philanthropic men and women everywhere to contribute to the cause.

Julius Hess spoke next: "I should like to emphasize the fact that we believe that those premature infants who have normal physiological development for their fetal age and show no inherited disease do not differ significantly as they grow older in weight or in mental development from their brothers and sisters or from other children." A perfect example of why he needed assistance from a showman.

Miss May Winter was trotted out as an example of "normal." Then the microphone was passed back to Martin. He was overwhelmed with gratitude. He said it. It was true. He had never had the good fortune to bring together forty graduates at once. And he was thrilled by the presence of leading doctors "who have come here for the purpose of convincing themselves that these babies are actually worth saving." Left unsaid: The presence of these doctors was proof at last that he wasn't crazy, or sleazy, or a quack.

Back in Atlantic City, Hildegarde received a shockingly tiny infant. The newspapers reported his name as Emanuel Sanfilipo and stated that he was born weighing nineteen ounces, in Hammonton, New Jersey. One paper boasted that while Canada had the Dionne quintuplets, Hammonton's baby was smaller than the littlest of them. When a state emergency

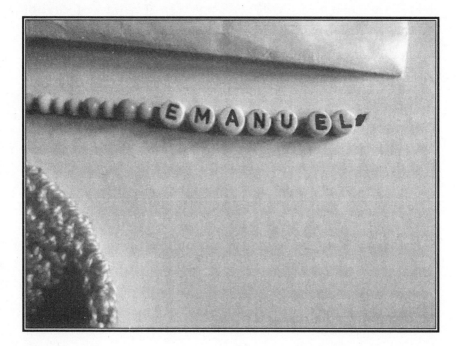

relief worker paid a visit to the home, she called her supervisor, who called a councilwoman, and they rushed the infant to the boardwalk.

Before long, Baby Emanuel was gaining. The problem was, he was born on August 7. In just a couple of weeks, the incubator station would close for the season.

Martin wanted Hildegarde to get on the train and carry the baby one thousand miles to the fair. The other babies in Atlantic City were ready to go home, but not Emanuel—he was under two pounds. The Century of Progress would run until November. And unlike the situation with the Dionne quintuplets—where, without his usual retinue, Martin's lack of medical training might have been exposed—he would have Julius on hand, plus Maye, Louise, and Hildegarde. Here was a nearly perfect opportunity.

The drama captivated the nation, as Martin knew it would. At noon on September 12, Hildegarde took Emanuel from the boardwalk in a heated carrier. At 2:50, they arrived at Pennsylvania Station in Manhattan. Next, they took a taxi crosstown to Grand Central. At 4:15 they boarded the train named the Twentieth Century. Martin, spending a fortune, reserved an entire car, heated to 80 degrees so Hildegarde could safely take the baby out and feed him.

Everybody waited. The AP News reported that "the flickering spark of life glimmered across half a Continent today . . ." The entire country breathed a sigh of relief when, at nine a.m. on September 13, the Twentieth Century rolled into Chicago with Baby Emanuel, alive.

Less than two weeks later, another impossibly small life arrived. This baby was born at Chicago's Cook County Hospital, weighing one pound, seven ounces, and like most newborns, it had already lost weight. Martin declared *this* was the littlest infant he had seen. Possibly, it was.

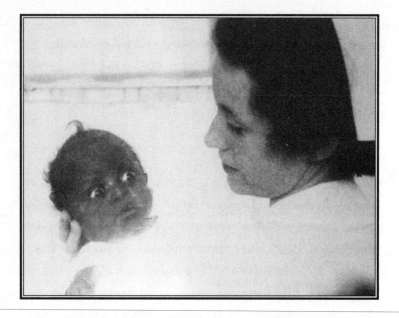

Louise Recht with a baby at the New York World's Fair.

"We cannot reveal the child's name," he said in a press release, "for that would be a breach of medical ethics. Later, if we are successful in our fight for the child's life we will be able to give out more information." He did not say whether the patient was a boy or a girl. The last line of the press release, which the fair sent out, was, "The child is colored."

The name was never revealed. Time and again, newspapers describing the shows in New York and Chicago mentioned "lots of Negro and Chinese babies." Children of color were photographed. But never was a nonwhite parent quoted—not even in the African American papers.

Come October, a cold snap forced the city into winter coats. Mobs of people bundled up to come for one last look. The Century of Progress made a modest profit—the fruit of a daring act of faith. In the infant incubators, some one hundred lives were saved.

But on November 1, just as the fair was shutting down, Baby Emanuel died.

In the winter of 1935, as the Deco pavilions crumbled under the wrecking balls, Herman Bundesen made his move, announcing a comprehensive plan to save the city's preemies. All Chicago hospitals were to receive protocols and would be required to fill out surveys that would make them aware of their deficiencies. The board of health purchased Hess beds to lend to hospitals and homes, opened free breast milk stations, and required all health professionals to report premature births immediately so a treatment plan could be made. A nurse who was specially trained at Sarah Morris would follow up until the infant weighed eight pounds. Already a frequent radio guest, Dr. Bundesen took a showbiz turn, arranging for a light to flash in a public space whenever a preemie died.

Chicago's citywide initiative was to become a model for the entire country.

Propaganda for preemies, indeed.

"MY LITTLE BROTHER"

A Sanfilippo family was listed in Hammonton, New Jersey. Almost eighty years earlier, the papers had spelled the baby's name "San-filipo," with one *p*. Contacting the family I'd found was like calling a number that was off by a digit and hoping the right person answered. I did it anyway. It worked.

Emanuel Sanfilippo, born in 1937, was named for his brother who'd died at the fair. "My parents never spoke about him, being very poor Italian immigrants," he wrote to me. But they kept the newspaper clippings, and the tiny knit hat, and the beaded necklace with his name on it. Emanuel sent me a photo with a handwritten note: "This hat belongs to Baby Emanuel born Aug. 7, 1934, was 19 oz. Born to Mary & Biagio Sanfilippo. My little brother." Those three words—*my little brother*—suffused with a quiet longing for a sibling never met; older, yet forever little.

He also sent copies of handwritten letters sent to the family by the Couneys. On August 23, 1934, Hildegarde wrote from the boardwalk to let Mary Sanfilippo know her son was doing well, encouraging her to keep her breast milk flowing. She closed with "Emanuel sends you all his love as well as big kisses." On August 30, she reported that the baby had gained thirty-five grams since her last letter. "He is a darling and I could just eat him up. He is very good, sleeps a lot & cries very little. He would like you to come & see him sometime." On September 6, she sent three dollars, round-trip bus fare for the Sanfilippos to come and see their baby. "He is getting cuter every day—sucks his thumb sometimes," she wrote.

The next communication was dated October 30, from Chicago. This time Hildegarde wrote that the baby had lost ground during the night. "The doctor has just been here to see him but he does not give up hope for him yet. There is still a chance even tho' it is only a small one."

A letter dated November 6 from the Right Reverend Monsignor William M. Foley of St. Ambrose Church certified that the baby was given a Christian burial according to the rites of the Catholic Church.

The final letter, dated November 8, was written by Maye:

My Dear Mrs. and Mr. Sanfilippo,

I wish to thank you for your prompt return of the consent. It came on Sunday and we called the undertaker at once and he arranged everything for us—and so very sweetly and nicely. Our little one was laid away on Tuesday morning, Nov. 6. Madame Recht, Hildegarde Couney and myself were present at the ceremony performed by the priest. I was wishing you might see it too. He had such a lovely white velvet casket with silver trimmings and a lovely crucifix. I'm sure you would have been more than satisfied. I'm sending you the papers and the note from the priest, also the necklace and his medal. And the first time we are in Atlantic City we will call on you.

With very best wishes for your [unclear] and your nice family believe me most sincerely.

Your friend,
Maye Couney

SORROW IN SEA GATE

New York, 1936

The Century of Progress should have marked the start of a golden passage in the Couneys' lives. But in February of '36, Maye was feeling ill. Isador was dying and wouldn't last through spring; he had a private nurse to tend to him. But Maye's condition was sudden, and urgent.

Martin, alarmed, must have put his connections to work. With his vast network, especially after Chicago, and his substantial wealth, he could have reached the best in any specialty with just a few calls.

On February 22, Maye was undergoing a craniotomy at the Neurological Institute in Manhattan. The surgeon cut open her skull. Somewhere in her brain was the story of her life. Thirty-five years with Martin. The day she first met him and the morning not long after, when a president was shot. The boardwalks and the nurseries. The salt and the blood. Whatever choices she regretted. The babies, always. Any secrets she would take to her grave.

Maye died on the table.

"LEAVE AS SOON AS YOU GET THIS"

The letter that came from Uncle Martin was blunt: *Get out, immediately.* Included were tickets and money and instructions. Pick up the baby and go. Don't stop to say good-bye. Don't pack. Get on the boat to New York, and I will take care of you.

Decades later, Martin's niece, Ilsa, and her husband, Dr. Alfred Ephraim, told the Gartners about leaving Berlin in 1937, and living in Sea Gate with their baby daughter until they could get their own place.

With Maye dead and Isador gone to his grave not three months later, Martin was grieving not only for them but also for his homeland. Better than most, he understood what was about to happen, and he intended to rescue as many Jews as he could. The U.S. government wasn't making it easy. The leaders of the American eugenics movement were persuasive with the State Department: No flood of Jews. Not here. To arrange for even one person required onerous paperwork, an affidavit swearing to accept financial responsibility, and proof of the means to do it. Which was still no guarantee of getting a visa.

Suddenly, Martin was everyone's "uncle" or "cousin," whether or not he knew them at all. He would meet them at the boat, and show them around New York in his chauffeured car, telling them where to shop, and what to do, and how to live in this country. Come Thanksgiving, the refugees were invited for dinner at his house. Most were soon able to fend for themselves, but he gave them money anyway, and plenty of it.

In the United States, no one kept records of affidavits signed. Ship manifests show at least eight people coming to Martin; Ilsa, who was there at the time, swore that the number was fifteen.

W hy do you want to know about my grand-uncle?" Ruth Freudenthal asked me. Her parents, Ilsa and Alfred, had died, but during the Day of Couney, it occurred to me that their baby, Ruth, was probably alive. She sounded not the least surprised that I'd found her, yet wondered why I wanted to write a book. Did I understand he was "more of a showman than a doctor"? After we talked for a while about her grand-uncle Martin, and Aunt Louise, and Aunt Hildegarde, she invited me to her home. "I'm the only one still alive who remembers them," she said wistfully.

It must feel odd to encounter a stranger who has been poking around your family, replaying your mother's voice on tape, visiting your relatives' graves, digging up records you hadn't thought to look for.

Ruth said that her mother was known as the family elephant; she remembered everything. "Whatever she said is true," Ruth told me emphatically. She was sorry her memory wasn't as good. But in fact, she recalled a lot, from getting caught standing on a table reaching for the crystal apples and pears in the chandelier at Sea Gate to playing with the midgets in Luna Park while visiting Uncle's concession. She was canny and smart (and her home was immaculate) in a way that made me perceive a family resemblance to the ghost who haunted me.

I showed her the picture I'd snapped of the house at the Couneys' address after I'd sweet-talked my way past the guard at the Sea Gate entrance. She wasn't sure it was the same. "It wasn't pink back then. I think it was gray," she said. "In the dining room, they had a huge glass table, which could probably seat sixteen to twenty people. Later, when he came to eat at our house, it had to be very special. Of course it had to be special anyway because he was my grand-uncle, but he was a gourmet."

Oddly, Martin wasn't in town during the first few months the Ephraims lived in his house; instead, he was off in Europe doing who knew what.* When he came back, he used his connections to help Ruth's father establish his dermatology practice. "Martin Couney was very wealthy," Ruth said several times. "He must have been very wealthy." That is, until the New York World's Fair. She showed me the Chinese cabinet he'd bought there while he was going broke; it sat in her living room now.

A s a child, Ruth would go to the Metropolitan Opera with Aunt Hildegarde; this was her birthday present every year, and she had to dress up and sit still. But the seats really belonged to a Sea Gate neighbor who had season tickets, and who went away each winter.

Hildegarde grew poorer as her health declined, and her body wasted away. "If I have a photograph of her in my wedding album, you'll see how thin she was," Ruth said, flipping through pages. "Everyone in all of these pictures is dead. It's really awful." And then there was Hildegarde, no longer husky but hauntingly gaunt, and close to death.

"She was buried in one of my dresses," Ruth said.

---

*Both Lawrence Gartner and I wondered whether he was involved in some kind of intelligence work. A half-dozen Freedom of Information Act requests turned up nothing, nor did an investigation by a Washington, D.C., researcher who specializes in these matters. Maybe he was simply a wealthy, well-connected, fluent, crafty widower traveling frequently to France before the war. Or not.

THE ONES WHO GOT AWAY

Norma Johnson and her twin brother, George, were born in July of 1937, weighing, respectively, two and a half and three pounds. When I called Norma, she didn't remember the name of the hospital, but she'd never forgotten the story about the patient next to her mother. The woman had given birth to premature twin boys. "The doctor said, 'The boys won't make it unless they are in an incubator. There's only one in the hospital, and we have a baby in it.' This mother said, 'I'm not putting them in Coney Island, no way,'" Norma told me. "The doctor said the same thing to my mother, and she said, 'Certainly.' The two boys died. It was very sad."

When we spoke, Norma (now Coe) and her brother were seventy-eight years old, with nine kids and thirteen grandchildren between them.

PLAYING WITH MATCHES

New York City, 1939

As the rain fell and the crowds stood shifting on their feet, Albert Einstein had a few words to say. It was April 30, 1939, opening day at the World of Tomorrow, New York City's world's fair. Its planners expected this fair to easily exceed Chicago's, in the rinky-dink middle of the country. Chicago was the Second City. New York was first, by far. Sixty different nations had pavilions. Germany fell out—but never mind. We had their wild-maned genius. In his thick German accent, Einstein said, "If Science, like Art, is to perform its mission truly and fully, its achievements must enter not only superficially but with their inner meaning, into the consciousness of people."

People were standing for hours on line at General Motors' Futurama. Inside, they rode in gliding chairs, witnessing a better world to come. Skyscrapers and highways, fourteen lanes across. On exiting, they proudly wore the button stating "I Have Seen the Future."

Chrysler presented automobile assembly, and Borden its milking machines, but RCA one-upped them with the television, magic in a box. In the pavilions, visitors sampled the Soviet Union, Poland, France, Japan, the smorgasbord of Sweden. Gussied up with Lifebuoy soap and hair pomade, they strained to see King George VI and Queen Elizabeth, making their maiden visit to the States. They gazed upon the Trylon and the Perisphere, the fair's iconic structures, and the sculptures on the walkways.

And having sopped up culture, having seen and heard and tasted the future and its commerce, they went where they really wanted to go: the Amusement Zone.

Built atop a swampy patch at the edge of the former garbage dump, the Amusement Zone was the place for naughty, bawdy fun. Futurama's designer, Norman Bel Geddes, contributed his Crystal Lassies, fronted by a buxom statue. A sign declared "Inside She's Real"—and for fifteen cents, you could see for yourself. Yes, there were wholesome aquatic shows and rides, but they were sprinkled in among Arctic Girls frozen naked in ice, and numerous other jiggle and strip joints—the occasional raid by the city's vice squad only a minor annoyance.

Then there was Salvador Dalí's Dream of Venus. The Surrealist's water show, in a building "bristling with appendages and cast in crepuscular light," was an erotic sore spot. The backers didn't care that the swimmers were topless. That was fine by them. They minded that that idiot Dalí envisioned some of the women with hideous fish heads, while anyone with an ounce of brains knew that you had to have pretty gals with mermaid tails. When the show opened (replete with bare-breasted women, warped clocks, lobsters, and inverted umbrellas—but nary a fish-headed swimmer), the artist allegedly air-dropped angry tracts over Manhattan before leaving the country in a fit of indignation.

Bizarre as the whole thing was, it wasn't as strange as sticking a pay-per-view NICU in back of the Parachute Jump, in a city that still lacked any kind of consistent, comprehensive care for preemies. But that's where Martin found himself. Despite the embrace of Julius Hess and Morris Fishbein, despite the well-known physicians now endorsing him in New York, despite the fact that the American Medical Association had honored him with a platinum watch, he was still an amusement.

B ack at the Century of Progress, the planners had gone out of their way to accommodate him. But in New York, relations with the concessions committee were fraying before the show opened. Martin had started early, writing in January of 1937 to express his interest in exhibiting, citing his enormous success in Chicago. He followed up with eight references, including Hess, Bundesen, and Fishbein. He sweetened his résumé, including not only Berlin and Paris but also Rio and Buenos Aires. Sometimes his list also included Mexico City, Montreal, and Moscow.

With permission, he dropped the names of Dr. Frederick Freed, from Bellevue's obstetrics department, and Dr. Thurman Givan, chief pediatrician at Cumberland Street Hospital and assistant chief of pediatrics at Long Island College Medical School. (Many years later, Thurman Givan would write that although Martin Couney was licensed in France, he didn't have the paperwork here, which is why he needed backup.) Both doctors asserted their willingness to take over in the event that Martin died during the course of the fair. By the time it started, he'd be seventy.

Hurdle number one was the committee member who objected to the exhibit because he'd conflated it with the two-headed dead-embryo show at the Century of Progress. Easily surmounted. The higher hurdle was money. Martin wanted this show to be grander than any he'd held before. And he planned to finance it entirely by himself, despite the fact that he'd never understood anything about money, aside from how to spend it generously. After the fair, he intended to give the building and all of its equipment to the City of New York—a permanent hospital, in memory of Maye.

THE STRANGE CASE OF DR. COUNEY

At first, he estimated initial expenses at $80,000. By February of 1938, that had already jumped to $100,000, and the committee wondered where the money was coming from. Martin ignored a request for a financial report.

The committee inquired around town. First National Bank & Trust Company of Coney Island said of Martin, "He enjoys a very fine reputation.... As he does not borrow from us we have no knowledge of his financial condition but from hearsay consider him in a position to undertake any obligation he may desire."

Dun & Bradstreet reported being unable to contact Dr. Couney. But two other banks responded favorably, and the committee surmised, based on what they'd cobbled together, that somehow or other, in various bank accounts, he had enough liquid assets.

He didn't. The marshy ground was a rat-infested mess, and everything was running over budget. He'd hired pricey Skidmore & Owings* to design the building. In addition to the nursery, the extravagant U-shaped structure included nine rooms of living quarters for himself, his nurses, wet nurses, chauffeur, and housekeeper; a courtyard with a garden; a glass-bricked area where babies who'd gained enough weight could bask in the sunlight; a room for presentations on baby care; and a special visiting room for doctors. By March of '39, it was clear it wouldn't be ready on time. An internal memo noted six carpenters "on a job that could easily stand twenty men." Martin, who'd hoped to pay in cash, was forced to sell critical stocks in a bad market.

Soon he was bickering about everything from smidgens of inches allowed for his outdoor sign to the officious insistence that he install an electric dishwasher. The nerve of these petty bureaucrats, telling him how

*Now Skidmore, Owings & Merrill, the firm later designed the John Hancock Center and the Sears (currently Willis) Tower in Chicago, and in this century, the "Freedom Tower" in New York City.

to run a nursery! As a matter of principle, he refused. (One paper quipped that he'd told them to "lay an egg.")

Then he became strangely upset by the requirement for a fire alarm. He, if anyone, knew the threat. Later that summer, Steeplechase Park would burn; the only reason his babies weren't there when it happened was that he had closed his other shows for the world's fair.

But the burden of having to manage without Maye was getting to him, and he couldn't afford to bleed another dime. He typed up a two-page letter arguing that a fire alarm was "absolutely unnecessary." The building was semi-fireproof; he had six extinguishers and a hose-reel connection inside. Three or four nurses were always awake, equipped with a telephone with four extensions. They had nightly fire drills. They set up baskets with hot-water bottles and blankets in case they needed to evacuate. His special ambulance was parked nearby, and he himself slept on the premises.

In conclusion, he wrote, "my nurses are strictly prohibited to smoke in the building and my babies do not play with matches. I hope you will see the justice of my claim and relieve me of the unnecessary expense." And then he went and did it. For the first time, he signed his name with an "M.D." at the end of it.

A couple of weeks past opening day, visitors were streaming into the finally ready concession. A thousand-pound reproduction of Andrea della Robbia's late-fifteenth-century bas-relief of a swaddled infant sat on the roof, and a sign declared that more than five million people had seen this show. Above the door: "All the World Loves a Baby."

A. J. Liebling came to write a profile for *The New Yorker*. "Everything I do is strict ethical," Martin stressed, still bothered by the rumors. And then he regaled Liebling with his stories: the beer hall songsters in Berlin; the hatbox baby in Omaha; the preemie who came to him wearing a necklace

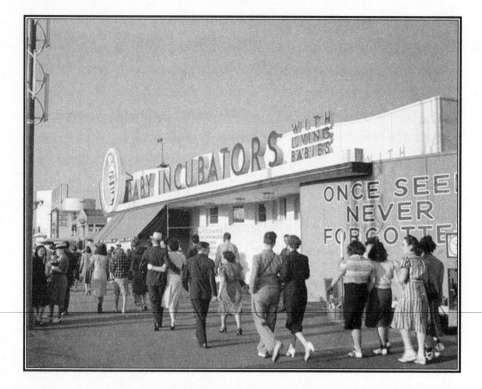

of garlic for strength; the Swedish grandma pulling a preemie through the leg of its father's trousers for luck; the Catholic babies wearing medals; the Jewish babies with a red thread to protect them against the evil eye. He also told Liebling that for Omaha, he'd taken the babies from Chicago (a feat that seems unlikely), while for Queen Victoria's Jubilee, he'd carried French orphans across the Channel (in wash baskets!), with the blessing of his mentor. (For *Family Circle*, he gilded the lily further, claiming that developing the incubator under Dr. Pierre Budin wasn't "intricate" work and "came from the heart, perhaps, as well as the head.")

In the Amusement Zone, men and women still dizzy from the thrill of their choice came through to ooh and aah and ask the usual loopy questions: "Are these the same babies from Chicago?" "How do they live in the gas stoves?"

Louise and Hildegarde were busy slipping diamond rings over wrists

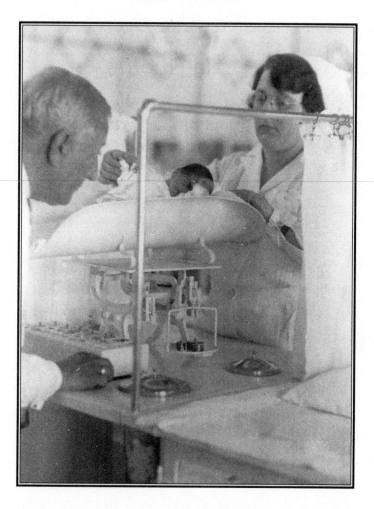

and smiling for the cameras. (Science entering the consciousness of the people, Dr. Einstein.) Hildegarde told a reporter, "I'd rather be helping my father with this work than doing anything else in the world." But Maye's absence must have been felt as a physical, daily ache.

Julius Hess paid a visit and left a letter for the guest book:

My Dear Martin,

Now that I cannot be with you in person may I be allowed to thank my "great teacher" in this wholly unsatisfactory way for your great contribution to me and the medical profession. Yours has not only been one of scientific leadership but equally important to progress a most ethical one in every respect, and you can look back on a life well spent.

May I add a word of deep and heartfelt remembrance for the years thru which I knew your Dear Wife and helpmate who for so many years was at your side. For Madame and Hildegarde my sentiments are those of deepest respect for them and their attainments as they so well know.

Again Martin may you live long and happily so that you may continue your great work on behalf of those so needing your help.

Your friend,
Julius H. Hess

But paper and ink are no substitute for having a friend in town who will see that you are treated with respect. In Chicago, he was a valued guest from the East, but here he was just the old man from Coney Island, past his prime. His posture was stooped, and he walked with a crook-handled cane, badly aged.

Martin had been confident that as soon as the show opened, he would recoup his investment. Soon it was obvious he was losing even more. Almost every concession was suffering, with the splashy exception of Billy Rose's Aquacade. The entire fair was sinking into debt. Admission was seventy-five cents—fifty percent more than the general admission in Chicago—and that was just to get in, before you spent a penny on the midway. People were still out of work. Yes, the crowds were thick—but nowhere near the planners' expectations. Worse for Martin, New Yorkers could have seen the incubators only the summer before at Coney Island, where the price had dropped to twenty cents. Why pay a quarter here?

One day a young woman strode up, eager to see the doctor. Her name was Lucille, and she was a nursing student at St. John's Episcopal Hospital in Brooklyn. Martin was easy to find. She walked over and told him, "I'm a baby of yours."

Visits like this were occurring with some frequency this summer. Sometimes it felt like the only recognition he was getting at this fair. He asked Lucille's last name and year of birth, then consulted a thick black book. There she was. *Lucille Conlin. 1920.* Father had brought her to Coney Island in a towel. Written off by a hospital. And look at her now, this healthy young lady, all of nineteen. "Yes, you are one of ours," he said, and hugged her, showed her around and showed her off.

A tall young man stood staring into an incubator as if he was willing the baby to live. Martin tapped him on the shoulder. "Is that your baby in there?"

"Yes." The familiar fear in the voice.

"You see this young lady?" Martin said. "She's one of our babies." The father regarded Lucille and then looked at his child and back at Lucille again. "She really is?" His daughter was so little—the size of his hand, perhaps. He must have been thinking that she would never grow up.

Before Lucille left, Martin made a note of where she went to school. The following year, he would send her a corsage when she earned her nurse's cap.

You don't know how much the help of the incubators meant to poor people like us," a twenty-three-year-old former telephone operator said to a reporter. "Dr. Couney even sent for our baby in his own ambulance with an incubator in it."

As always, a physician was tucked in behind the scenes. Moe Goldstein was young. He had gone to medical school with Morris Fishbein's son-in-law, then finished a fellowship at the Mayo Clinic, returning home to open a pediatric practice in Queens. But business was slow. And here was a fascinating job, suggested to him by the powerful editor of the country's most prestigious medical journal. Who would turn that down? As far as Moe could tell, his boss was a doctor, but somehow lacked a license in New York—or something like that. He could never get a straight answer. And it didn't really matter.

Every evening, Moe would come and examine the babies, and stay and eat a good meal and have a good drink and pass the time with Martin. He thoroughly enjoyed his host. And he was in awe of Madame. She knew how to do things, like nasal feeding, that no one had taught him in medical school or at the Mayo Clinic. He was learning skills that would put him ahead in his fledgling practice. Plus, these babies would need a pediatrician after the fair, and he was the logical choice.

While he was at it, he helped the gals from the jiggle joint next door. Most of them were mothers with new babies. That's who had big breasts. They simply needed money. They brought him their babies when they were sick, and he took care of them.

Moe was aware that the concession was doing something exceptional. Babies under three pounds should have had something like a 90 percent mortality rate, yet almost all of them were being saved. Martin had put him in charge of keeping records. The tiniest went in Hess beds, with oxygen lids, while the rest went in Martin's sleeping-beauty machines. Some of those babies got a little oxygen too. But not much.

Late in his life, Moe would say, "Dr. Hess copied a good deal of Dr. Couney's system" from the Chicago fair. He also remembered the chauffeured ambulance that far preceded New York City's premature transport system.

The only thing not to Moe's liking that summer was Hildegarde. He was certain the boss's daughter had a crush on him, and he found her unappealing.

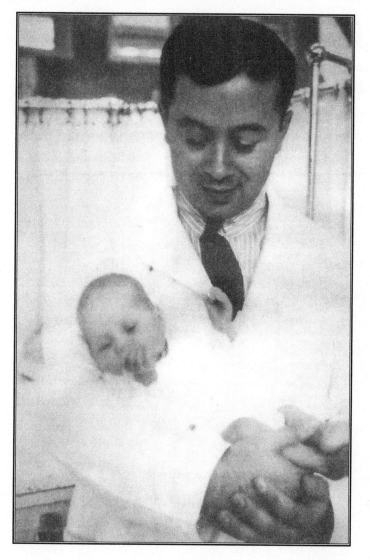

Dr. Moe Goldstein.

All that summer and the next, a team of doctors came from Yale to study the "fetal infants." Drs. Arnold Gesell and Catherine Amatruda were trying to understand the beginnings of visual and auditory awareness, manual grasp, a response to a smile—the ignition of the human mind. Martin and Louise ("Madame" to them) went out of their way to accommodate them.

Quietly, out of view of the crowd, Gesell and Amatruda measured, observed, and, with a cameraman, took photos, and shot grainy, silent film.

The Embryology of Behavior, considered a medical classic, was published in 1945. In some of the photos the infants are nude. Without their prince and princess swaddling, their ribbons, their blankets, their baby-doll caps, they are big-headed and frog-legged, almost amphibian.

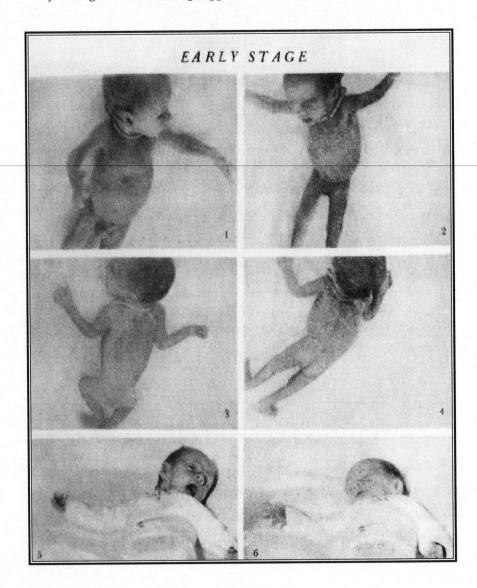

EARLY STAGE

Martin was ever jolly in public, but behind the scenes, his relations with the administration were increasingly testy. He griped about the "sketchily dressed" women outside the Enchanted Forest and the Kootch Show in the Canine Capers building. They hit back with a medical complaint. Why had someone named Moe Goldstein signed a death certificate? Who was this person, anyway? Might they remind the doctor that he was obliged to comply with the laws, statutes, ordinances, rules, and regulations of the government of the City and State of New York and of the United States? The letter further enjoined him to permit an inspection by the fair's Dr. John Grimley—the dishwasher enthusiast, with whom he'd clashed before—and to report to *him* rather than directly to his health department contact. This particular dust-up settled down after Martin assured them that his assistant, Moe Goldstein, had a license.

But the money problems worsened. By July, Martin was threatening to quit, unless the Comptroller's Office could ease the terms of a loan it had made. He couldn't, and wouldn't, reduce personnel or skimp on care. The fair agreed to cut him a break. But by the season's end, around the time Germany invaded Poland, Martin's accounts were running bloody red.

VISION AND HINDSIGHT

Katherine Ashe Meyer e-mailed to tell me she'd seen my post on a 1939 New York World's Fair forum: "I would love to talk to you and I am also interested if you have heard from any of the other 'babies.'" She'd kept her autographed glossy of Martin Couney, and a photo of Moe Goldstein holding her, and her parents' free-admission passes.

Kathy was born on July 19, around the time Martin was threatening to close up shop. "My mother was skinny as a rail, and when my parents got to the hospital, they said, 'What are you here for?' She said, 'I'm going to have a baby,' and they said, 'You've got to be kidding.'" Born two months early, Kathy weighed three pounds, four ounces.

New York Hospital was among the city's most advanced, and it had an incubator for her—at a cost that was out of reach. "My father went to them and said, 'This is going to cost me a fortune. I'm not working, I just bought a house in Queens, and I've got a three-year-old. What do I do?' They said, 'We'll put you on a payment plan.' My father said, 'I really can't do that.' And then the pediatrician said, 'You know, one of my friends has a preemie show at the World's Fair, why don't we see if we can get her in?'"

Kathy's parents—unlike most of the women I spoke with—were happy to talk to her about the show. "They were so proud of it," she said. "My

The visitor passes for Katherine Meyer's parents were labeled "concessionaire." The couple also kept souvenir photos of the King and Queen of England.

mother expressed her milk and my father took it over every day. They thought it was the best thing in the world."

Nine years later, her parents got a call from New York Hospital, asking them to bring her for an exam. "They said to my father, 'There is something we don't understand. All the babies that were in our incubators are going blind—but your baby's eyes are good.'"

WHO WILL SAVE YOU NOW?

New York City, 1940

T he incubator concession had burned through more than $100,000
in operating expenses during the fair's first season—$3,000 in laun-
dry alone, plus thirty people on salary (nurses, wet nurses, lecturers,
ticket takers, kitchen help). Moe was never paid—he was given a watch
instead, not that he minded. But receipts, minus the fair's cut, were nowhere near enough to break even.

The administration weighed its options. Privately, they discussed what
it would cost to move the concession to the Science and Education Wing
of the Medical and Public Health Building—but decided not to do it. At
the same time, an official wrote to the Smith Incubator Corporation in
Ohio, asking if *they* wanted the show for 1940. Not a chance.

With his contract not renewed by March, Martin's debt to the fair corporation was almost $10,000. In order to open again, he would need to
mortgage his house, borrow from friends, ask contractors to wait to be
paid, and defer his space rental charges. He'd mistaken a previous "deferred"
debt for one that was waived, and he pleaded to have it forgiven. Also, he
asked, as a courtesy, could they please turn the water back on?

Behind closed doors, the reaction was exasperation. Patronizing. "As you perhaps know, Dr. Couney is well into his 80s [*sic*], rather feeble and prone to misunderstanding," read one internal note. "What he actually needs is a business manager to take care of all financial affairs. His late wife was very successful in handling such matters, but since her death, he is lost when it comes to money matters. His operation last year was not at all successful and his statement is a jumble of figures. . . . There is no degree of certainty as to their exactness without some sort of an examination of his books which would be an unnecessary expense."

In the end, they agreed on a plan where his debt would be paid through his weekly receipts, and he opened up again.

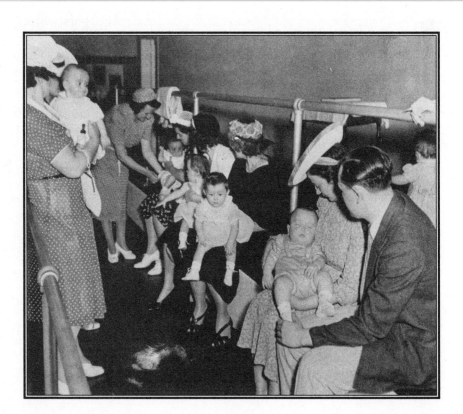

No matter what he lost, he wouldn't pass up a chance to make propaganda. The previous fall, when Julius was in town, he'd hosted a gala dinner. Each week, the nurse whose babies gained the most weight won a prize, such as nylon hosiery. Come June, he threw a reunion for the class of '39, and once again handed out silver cups. In July, he entertained Morris Fishbein's son, Justin, visiting from out of town. And as the season came to end, he invited a tableful of prominent pediatricians to eat and drink and smoke cigars and listen to Moe Goldstein present the concession's results: proof they had saved more than 90 percent of their patients.

On November 9, 1940, a single paragraph about Martin Couney's incubators appeared in Morris Fishbein's *Journal of the American Medical Association*—the first and only time Couney's name would appear in those pages.

Away from the crowds and the parents and the feted special guests, Moe saw Martin crying. A pall had fallen over the fair, and no one could ignore it, no matter how they tried. Ten of the foreign nations hadn't come back, including the Soviet Union. Poland's pavilion was draped in black; Finland's closed mid-season. The night that Germany invaded France, Moe was with his boss, who was inconsolable.

Martin was also losing every dollar he and Maye had ever earned, forced to keep begging the fair's administration. Unless they reduced the cut they had taken toward his debt, he wouldn't be able to pay the nurses' salaries. The moneymen relented and gave him an allowance. But he was almost seventy-one, and he knew he was in a position from which he could never recover. At night, with the babies of 1940 baking in their ovens—to inherit what kind of a world?—he would go to his private garden to weep.

The World of Tomorrow closed on October 27, 1940, a financial disaster for almost everyone involved. As for Martin's state-of-the art lifesaving equipment, the city didn't want it.

WINTER

artin and Louise could not afford to retire. Back in Luna Park, with
Coney Island's luster faded and rubbed away, admission was down
to fifteen cents. In Atlantic City, entrance was still by donation.
This was no way to regain a lost fortune. Still, there were babies to save.

Carol Boyce was born at Atlantic City Hospital on June 19, 1942, weighing just over four pounds. Not so tiny, really, for a preemie, but upon hearing the news, her grandmother bought a white dress for her "just in case."

Carol Boyce Heinisch was living in Absecon, New Jersey, when I reached
her. At seventy-three, she worked part-time as a legal assistant. With
her keen interest in local history, she knew about the plaque that Lawrence Gartner put up in 1971. Originally affixed to the Holiday Inn that
stood on the former site of the show, it went to Atlantic City's historical
museum when the hotel came down, and now it was sitting tarnished.
Carol had newspaper clippings and photos for me. And I had her mother's
voice, recorded forty-five years earlier. In the recording, the late Betty
Boyce fondly remembered "Aunt Louise" and Hildegarde. She met Martin
only once. "He had the ability to put you at ease right away," she said. "It

was like, maybe your child was half-dead, but no problem. Everything will turn out fine."

C ome winter, with the boardwalk desolate and snow falling over the ocean, with all the young men gone to war, Martin, Louise, and Hildegarde retreated to a lonely life. Sea Gate was quiet. The wealthy neighbors spent the frozen months in warmer places. For company, Martin had his poodles. Louise kept a little Pekingese so mean you couldn't touch it.

A visitor was a treat. Dr. Frederick Freed, disappointed at being rejected by the army, joined the Couneys for Christmas in 1942. Years later, Moe Goldstein, home from the war, stopped by Sea Gate to chat. "When they first discovered retrolental fibroplasia, Dr. Couney and I used to sit and talk," he would tell Lawrence Gartner. "He used to say, 'I don't know.

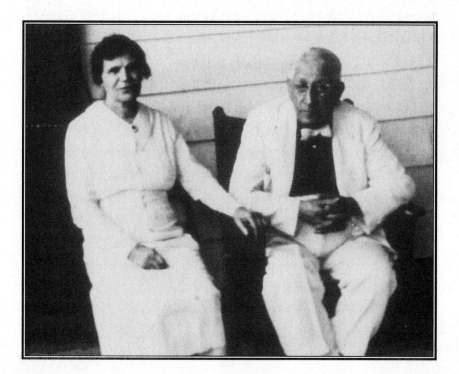

I never saw any in mine. I took care of thousands of them, and none of my babies were ever blind.'" The answer was that his machines never had enough oxygen to do that kind of damage, especially because the nurses kept taking the babies out. But Martin wouldn't live to know it.

Sometimes, toward the end of his life, when he got his mail, he would find a check—a gift from Julius Hess or Thurman Givan, or another of his medical friends. It pained him to accept it, but he had to. Already, the deed to the house had passed to Hildegarde; she would need to sell it the minute he died.

"In the last year, he was very bad, financially very bad," his niece, Ilsa, said. "But even in the last few weeks, he wouldn't have hesitated to invite you out for dinner."

Every year, when the weather turned, the babies went home to their parents. They learned to crawl and they went to school and they walked in caps and gowns. They went to work in offices and factories and hospitals and boardrooms. They went to fight a war and then another. They married. They went to town in new cars. They threw away their hats. They walked around in new clothes that didn't require an iron. They walked their children down the aisle. The sat in front of their televisions and watched a man walk on the moon. They took their children's children to the ocean. They bought a new computer and got someone young to help. Some of them went to their graves, but others stepped out of one century and into the next, run on technology that no one, not even Einstein, could have foreseen. They had their knees replaced. They Skyped. They Googled the man who had saved their lives seventy, eighty, ninety years earlier, but all they could find were the things he had said.

In 1943, Cornell New York Hospital opened the city's first dedicated premature infant station. That same year, Dr. Martin Couney closed his show for the final time. He said his work was done.

EPILOGUE

A cool, end-of-September breeze was blowing through New York. At 8:40 that morning, the plane carrying Pope Francis took off from JFK, ending a forty-hour visit that had gridlocked Manhattan and somehow bathed the city in a fleeting sweet mood.

Uptown at Morgan Stanley Children's Hospital of New York-Presbyterian, where William Silverman trained a generation of doctors, the treatment of preemies proceeded in its never-ending cycle. Intubated infants drew in exquisitely calibrated doses of oxygen or were assisted in their breathing by continuous positive airway pressure (CPAP). Food flowed through tubes into their mouths or noses, and medication dripped into their bandaged bodies intravenously.

The doctors and nurses on the floor are among the best in the world. Currently in charge is Richard A. Polin, M.D., William T. Speck Professor of Pediatrics, College of Physicians and Surgeons, Columbia University, and director of the Division of Neonatology. He maintains that skilled nursing, hand hygiene, and the use of breast milk are all important—all things that Martin Couney stressed way back when, along with loving touch. Parental bonding, which has replaced the limited-visitation, hands-off approach, is also encouraged and considered important.

On that late-September day, as happened every day on Dr. Polin's ward, mothers and fathers sat incubator-side or cradled their tiny newborns, holding them gently so as not to disturb the wires connected to monitors and the tubes delivering sustenance, singing softly, some of them, whispering, "I love you."

Out at Coney Island, end-of-season stragglers sauntered down the new, improved boardwalk, which had replaced the splintery wood destroyed by Hurricane Sandy. They waded in their rolled-up pants into the chilly Atlantic and wandered up the beach toward the concessions. A couple of blocks inland, the residents of Luna Park Building 2 were sleeping in or going about their usual Saturday business, most of them unaware that their apartment complex sat on the site of an incubator sideshow.

Up the parkway twenty-some miles, in Long Beach, Long Island, Barbara Horn was preparing to retrieve her ninety-five-year-old mother, Lucille, from a nursing facility. The occasion was a reunion of Martin Couney's babies.

The last baby homecoming was held in 1940 at the World of Tomorrow, solely for the class of '39. This twenty-first-century gathering—come one, come all—grew out of months of planning and logistics, after Barbara Gerber (class of '34), told me she was coming in to visit from California. She was staying in Long Beach, close to our meeting place at Barbara Horn's apartment. By six that morning, Kathy Meyer ('39) was en route from Connecticut. Her husband was ill, and her plans involved a relay of trains and family arrangements, but she was determined. "I missed the reunion in 1940 because I got sick," she said. "I don't want to miss this one." Betty Heinisch ('42) was traveling 150 miles from Absecon, near Atlantic City. Beth Allen ('41) needed a ride from suburban New Jersey, so I'd be picking her up and we'd make the hour-plus drive together.

Had Martin Couney been in charge, today's luncheon would have been

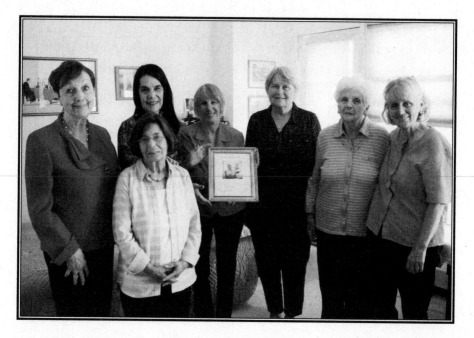

September 26, 2015: Carol Heinisch, Barbara Gerber, Dawn Raffel, Beth Allen (holding a photo of Dr. Couney), Katherine Meyer, Lucille Horn, and her daughter Barbara Horn.

over-the-top: *Platinum cups for everyone, forget about the cost!* Instead, it was I who had planned things. The best I could do was order a cake. "Write 'Happy Reunion' on it," I told the baker.

Martin Couney's driving was famously atrocious. Mine is not much better. Put me on a freeway with vehicles gunning from thirty directions and signage designed by sadists, and I freak. Now Beth Allen was in the car, along with the cake and the paper plates and the forks and the knives rattling in the back. *Please, don't let me kill her,* I prayed, as we scrambled through honking traffic.

Life is full of unexpected outcomes. I got us to Long Beach without even getting lost.

One by one the women arrived, in their black slacks and their colorful tops—red and green and speckled blue. They greeted one another not as strangers but as friends who had a deep-as-bones connection. In Barbara Horn's small living room, their questions overlapped: "Were you a twin too?" "How much did you weigh at birth?" "How long were you on the boardwalk?" "Did anyone other than Martin Couney think that you would live?" Among them, they had celebrated 399 birthdays. Glossy autographed photos of Uncle Martin and Aunt Louise emerged from tote bags, along with yellowing newspaper clippings and tiny ID bracelets with names spelled out in beads. Kathy had her silver cup; she'd missed the reunion, but Martin had sent it to her mother anyway. Out on the porch, the women posed for photographs together, with the ocean in the background, the wind in their hair.

Lucille Conlin Horn, class of 1920, was the oldest. She had grown frailer in the six months since I'd first met her. Back then, her short-term memory had already lost its rooting, but her grasp of the distant past was firm. Her beauty was serene and her blue eyes filled with light. "They said I would never live a day," she had said with evident pleasure in her graveled voice. She had told me the story of her birth, of her father taking her to the sideshow in a towel, and about the day she visited Martin Couney at the World of Tomorrow. In the end, she did not become a nurse; she married and had five children.

Now Lucille had moved from her daughter's apartment to a nearby nursing home. Unsteady on her feet and slightly lost, she needed prompting, yet she was clearly happy to be there. As she remembered Martin Couney, her confusion seemed to lift. One more time she recalled the day at the fair, before the war, when she, a young woman, met the man who saved her.

At ninety-five, Lucille had the kind of radiant grace that very old people sometimes have when everything inessential falls away. "He was a very nice man," she said, folding her hands in her lap.

r. Martin A. Couney died on March 1, 1950, and was buried with his wife, Maye, at Cypress Hills Cemetery in Brooklyn. Although the book of records he kept has never been found, every estimate puts the number of children whose lives he saved at between 6,500 and 7,000. There is nothing at his grave to indicate that he did anything of note.

Madame Amelie Louise Recht died the year after her boss, in the spring of 1951. She is buried in Holy Cross Cemetery.

Hildegarde Couney continued to work as a nurse but suffered for years from poor health. She never married or had children. In 1956 she was found dead in her Brooklyn apartment, and she was buried with "Aunt Louise." She was forty-nine.

Dr. Julius Hess continued to treat and fight for preemies until his death in 1955. He is widely credited as the father of American neonatology.

Lucille Marion Conlin Horn died on February 9, 2017, at the age of ninety-six. She is buried with her twin sister, who lived for twenty minutes.

ACKNOWLEDGMENTS

The long list of people I need to thank begins with Dr. Lawrence Gartner, who generously shared his research and insights, not only during the Day of Couney but at several other points in the course of writing this book. Dr. Carol Gartner also contributed to the research and discussion. Without them, this book would have been greatly diminished, and many more puzzles would have remained unsolved.

The work of the original Couney buffs, in particular the late Dr. William Silverman and the late Dr. L. Joseph Butterfield, was crucial. Other Couney sleuths, including those who joined in the 1990s, are: Dr. Jeffrey P. Baker, Dr. Julia Whitefield, Dr. Leonore Ballowitz, Dr. Thomas E. Cone, Dr. Murdina M. Desmond, Dr. Lula O. Lubchenco, Dr. Russell A. Nelson, Dr. O. Ward Swamer, and Dr. Paul L. Toubas. I'd also like to cite Dr. Ray Duncan, webmaster at Neonatology.org, for keeping so much information accessible, and for pointing me in the right direction more than once.

Dr. Gerald Oppenheimer, professor of clinical sociomedical sciences at the Mailman School of Public Health at Columbia University, studied Martin Couney in the process of writing an excellent history of the beginnings of neonatal public health policy. He took the time to discuss not only his research but also this book and the shape it would take. It was he who first suggested that I carefully examine midway entertainment, including the treatment of "freaks," indigenous peoples, and even animals.

Ruth Freudenthal, Martin Couney's grandniece, welcomed me into her home and shared her past in a way that deepened my understanding of this remarkable family. Thank you.

While conducting my research, I had the good fortune of being an Allen Scholar at the New York Public Library, which offered space to write and a wealth of archival resources. The Brooke Russell Astor Rare Manuscript Division was a godsend, as were the genealogy and map divisions. In particular, I want to acknowledge Amanda Seigel in the Dorot Jewish Division, and Carolyn Broomhead and Melanie Locay, who run the Allen Scholar program, offering constant support and keeping everyone sane.

The Coney Island Museum sparked this quest, and I extend gratitude to artistic director Dick Zigun and to Jay Singer; the latter helped me sort out exactly where Martin Couney's concession stood, and clued me in to the odd fact that in 1888, arriving immigrants' first sighting of the New World was the Elephant Hotel. Thanks, too, to Charles Denson at the Coney Island History Project.

At the Queens Museum, Richard J. Lee helped me sift through images of the New York World's Fair and connected me to collectors, including Paul Brigandi, who in turn led me to George C. Tilyou III.

Arlene Shaner, reference librarian at the New York Academy of Medicine, fielded multiple long-shot requests and offered me access to, among other things, a history of New York's Sloane Hospital, and Arnold Gesell and Catherine Strunk Amatruda's *Embryology of Behavior*, filled with images taken at Martin Couney's show. The New-York Historical Society's extensive collection of world's fair clippings and memorabilia helped put events in perspective. Michael Simonson, archivist at the Leo Baeck Institute, shed some light on Martin Couney's hometown, Krotoschin.

In Chicago, I found initial inspiration at the Chicago Historical Society. The records of Julius Hess and Evelyn Lundeen, along with press releases from the Century of Progress, were to be found at the Regenstein Library at the University of Chicago, while the administrative records of the Century of Progress are held by the Richard J. Daly Library at the University of Illinois in Chicago; the librarians and staff at both institutions were extremely generous in their assistance. Sarah Kirby also helped with preliminary research and Eliot Fackler tracked down photos in Chicago.

The archives at the American Academy of Pediatrics, outside Chicago, hold many of the Couney buffs' records. My thanks to Veronica Booth for arranging for my visit, which included the pleasure of seeing rare video footage of the incubator doctor himself. Allison Seagram provided additional assistance.

Cynthia Van Ness, director of Library and Archives at the Buffalo History Museum, went the extra mile to help me find information about the Pan-American Exposition and the assassination of William McKinley, sending the microfiche of Dr. Matthew Mann's scrapbooks downstate so I could find his century-old ticket to the incubator show. Elaine Mosher, library coordinator and assistant research professor of pediatrics at Women & Children's Hospital of Buffalo, provided me with information about the incubators themselves and gamely conducted a search to see whether any of Dr. Couney's machines might still be somewhere on the premises (sadly, not).

Valuable intel about Martin Couney's activities in Omaha came from the Omaha Public Library and the Omaha Historical Society. Timothy Schaffert, whose novel *The Swan Gondola* is set at the Trans-Mississippi Exposition, provided perspective.

Finding the original, signed naturalization papers for "Martin A. Coney" was a yearlong goose chase through the files of the National Archives, as well as various courts in Omaha. Thank you to Vikki Henry, a research volunteer at the Greater Omaha Genealogical Society, who finally found them.

Molly Kodner, archivist at the Missouri History Museum Library and Research Center, made it possible for me to get copies of transcripts and correspondence crucial to understanding the debacle at the St. Louis World's Fair; she also provided a copy of Dr. John Zahorsky's book.

Lorna Kirwin at the Bancroft Library, at the University of California at Berkeley, helped me access the records of the 1915 San Francisco World's Fair. Quentin Robinson at the Tippecanoe County Historical Association Library and Archives uncovered information about Maye Couney's mother, including the contents of her will. Stephen R. Wilk brought to my attention to Martin Couney's concession in Revere, Massachussetts.

Many other individuals helped me find "babies" and information. Carrie Brown, the author of *The Hatbox Baby*, a moving novel based on a fictional Dr. Couney, connected me with Lucille Horn, for which I am eternally grateful. Michael P. Onorato, an author and historian who wrote the epilogue for the reissue of Edo McCullough's *Good Old Coney Island* published in 2000, clarified for me that Martin Couney was at Steeplechase, not just Dreamland and Luna Park.

Thank you to Steven Pressman, whose book *50 Children: One Ordinary American Couple's Extraordinary Rescue Mission into the Heart of Nazi Germany* sheds light on the difficulty faced by Jews trying to escape Hitler's Germany. Steven connected me with Ron Coleman, reference librarian at the United States Holocaust Memorial Museum, who helped me find records of some of the people who came to the United States with Martin Couney as their connection.

Richard Polin, M.D., director of neonatology at New York-Presbyterian Morgan Stanley Children's Hospital, graciously gave me a tour of the NICU so that I could see the most cutting-edge treatment available today, and answered my layperson's questions.

My gratitude to the "babies" knows no bounds: Beth Allen, the late Lucille Horn (and her daughter Barbara Horn), Katherine Ashe Meyer, Barbara Gerber, Carol Heinisch, Norma Coe, Jean Harrison, and Jane Umbarger—you are the heart of this book.

Thank you to Emanuel San Filippo for sharing treasured mementos of his brother, to Ryna Appleton Segal for taking the time to talk with me about her mother's remarkable life, and to Nedra Justice and Joy (Musselwhite) Aimetti for providing their families' stories.

Nanette Varian always seemed to see relevant clippings before I did; I am lucky to have a friend who is a gifted investigator. Brendan Raffel Evers conducted a couple of reconnaissance missions—in particular, retrieving the deed to the Couneys' house. Among the many who made suggestions, served as a sounding board, or offered a strong arm pulling me back from the ledge: Cherie Raffel, Terese Svoboda, Tracy Young, Cindy Handler, Diane DeSanders, Pamela Ryder, Erika Goldman, Judy Sternlight, Bonnie Friedman, Charles Salzberg, Ona Gritz, Etta Jacob, and Joyce Raffel (who provided me with my grandmother's souvenirs from the Century of Progress). Thanks, as always, to Gordon Lish. I'm indebted to "the salon": Catherine Woodard, Helen Klein Ross, Chip Brown, Kate Walbert, Will Blythe, Claudia Burbank, and the rest of rotating gang.

My extraordinary agent, Melanie Jackson, believed in this book from the outset—wait, let's go back. She also believed in my previous books from the outset. For this endeavor, she offered critical encouragement and suggestions countless times along the way. "This book couldn't have happened without her" is a well-worn cliché, but in this case, it's entirely true.

My editors patiently waded through multiple drafts: Thank you to David Rosenthal for beginning this journey and to Stephen Morrow, who understood exactly what I needed to do to complete it, helping me make this a far better book. I'd also like to thank Katie Zaborsky and Madeline Newquist, as well as Kathleen Go, Anna Jardine, Loren Jaggers, and the rest of the publishing team.

Above all, I am eternally thankful to my husband, Michael Evers, and our sons, Brendan and Sean, for allowing Martin Couney to move in with our family and make himself at home for several years. And finally, thank you to Pierre the rescue terrier for waiting patiently while I wrote and reminding me to get up and play once in a while.

NOTES

Prologue: Breath

1 **The pains came too early:** Lucille Conlin Horn (the baby) and her daughter Barbara Horn, interview with the author, April 12, 2015. The account of the birth, including the dialogue with the obstetrician, is from this interview.

1 **drew breath for twenty minutes:** Barbara Horn, interview with the author, February 14, 2017.

"All the World Loves a Baby"

5 **the cops shot down John Dillinger:** "Kill Dillinger Here," *Chicago Tribune*, July 23, 1934 (reporting the previous day's shooting), p. 1.

5 **hottest day ever on record:** National Weather Service, http://www.weather.gov/lot /Chicago_Temperature_Records; "Break in Heat Due Tonight; Airport 109," *Chicago Tribune*, July 24, 1934, p. 1. The record remains unbroken as of this writing.

5 **people fled to the beaches:** Tom Skilling, "Baked City: Chicago's Hottest Week Occurred July 19–25, 1934," *Chicago Tribune*, July 19, 2009, p. I-35.

6 **a written instruction not to conduct:** Infant incubator homecoming script for July 25, 1934, Century of Progress International Exposition Scrapbook, Crerar Ms 227, Special Collections Research Center, University of Chicago Library.

6 **the midget wedding:** "Midget City News, Summer 1934," p. 13, Century of Progress International Exposition Scrapbook, Crerar Ms 227, Special Collections Research Center, University of Chicago Library. The wedding took place on July 13, 1934.

9 **forty-two "lusty-lunged boys and girls":** Press release, July 18, 1934, Century of Progress International Exposition Press Releases July 16–31, Crerar Ms 225, Special Collections Research Center, University of Chicago Library.

9 **Singles, twins . . . Miss May Winter:** Press release, July 24, 1934, Century of Progress International Exposition Press Releases July 16–31. The press release is written in past tense but was released the day before the reunion.

9 **Anyone who'd ever bought a pickle in Atlantic City:** The Heinz Pickle Pier was a major attraction. For an excellent history of Atlantic City's historic boardwalk, see Vicki Gold Levi, Lee Eisenberg, Rod Kennedy, and Susan Subtle, *Atlantic City: 125 Years of Ocean Madness* (New York: C. N. Potter, 1979).

10 **Excepting some members of the medical establishment:** For example, in a letter dated November 15, 1979, George Waddell, M.D., wrote to William Silverman, M.D., about his experience touring the 1934 show with residents from the University of Chicago Clinics. Waddell stated that he'd been unaware that Couney had been putting on shows for more than thirty years. He also wrote that while the doctors were impressed with the incubators, which were "far better" than any they'd seen in their short experience, they also felt "a little uneasy in the belief that there was something unethical about the whole show." His letter encapsulates the ambivalence of many physicians; he added, "I like to think that the Isolette in some way came into being because of the example of Dr. Couney's incubator." Newborn Medicine History Collection, Pediatric History Center, American Academy of Pediatrics.

10 **The script included Dr. Julius Hess ... And Dr. Herman Bundesen:** Infant incubator homecoming script for July 25, 1934, Century of Progress International Exposition Scrapbook.

10 **a man who was known to be:** Dr. Herman Bundesen's fondness for publicity is detailed in Gerald Oppenheimer, "Prematurity as a Public Health Problem: US Policy from the 1920s to the 1960s," *American Journal of Public Health* 86, no. 6 (June 1996), pp. 870–878. In 1933 alone, Dr. Bundesen was on the radio 435 times.

10 **air-conditioned:** "Babies, Babies, and Babies at World's Fair: Incubator Kiddies Will Be on Exhibit," *Chicago Tribune*, June 5, 1932, p. 20.

11 **Over in the Great Hall within the Hall of Science:** For a complete description, see Harry H. Laughlin (Eugenics Record Office, Carnegie Institution of Washington, Cold Spring Harbor, Long Island, New York), "The Eugenics Exhibit at Chicago: A Description of the Wall-Panel Survey of Eugenics Exhibited in the Hall of Science, Century of Progress Exposition, Chicago, 1933–34," *The Journal of Heredity* 26, no. 4 (April 1935), pp. 155–162. The previous issue of the journal (March 1935) states on its cover that the coming issue will include reporting of the first world's fair to recognize "the science and art of applying heredity to human affairs."

11 **pickled fetuses for public edification:** *Medical Science Exhibits*, 1934. University of Illinois at Chicago, University Library Special Collections, Century of Progress records, Box 24, folder 326, pp. 114–116.

11 **What he lacked in height:** Most of his records place Martin Couney at about five-seven or five-eight.

13 **Hiya, Doc, where'dja get the eggs?:** Multiple newspapers mention this and other ridiculous questions; see also Oliver Pilat and Jo Ranson, *Sodom by the Sea: An Affectionate History of Coney Island* (Garden City, NY: Doubleday, Doran, 1941), p. 198.

13 **Today, they were serving an elegant luncheon:** Press release, July 18, 1934, Century of Progress International Exposition Press Releases July 16–31.

13 **multiple seatings at dinner:** Letter from Barbara Fishbein Friedell to Richard F. Snow, 1981 (exact date unknown), Newborn Medicine History Collection, Pediatric History Center, American Academy of Pediatrics.

13 **here in Chicago, they rarely left the fairgrounds:** Friedell distinctly recalls this, although there is an element of doubt. The *Chicago Tribune* noted that in early August of

the previous year, Dr. Couney was so irritated by the noise from Harry's New York Bar across the way that he'd begun decamping to a "swanky" hotel each night at ten p.m. "Sauce for the Goose," *Chicago Tribune*, August 6, 1933, p. F1.

14 **Martin loved to cook . . . His palate was discerning:** Ruth Freudenthal (Couney's grandniece), interview with the author, August 18, 2015. In a 1939 newspaper, Martin Couney is quoted as saying, "I can do more with a soupbone than most Americans can do with steak." Otherwise undated, unidentified clipping, Newborn Medicine History Collection, Pediatric History Center, American Academy of Pediatrics.

15 **Julius and Clara Hess were often . . .** *les escargots:* Letter from Friedell to Snow.

15 **his personal story, which he continued to perfect:** Martin Couney told versions of this story to numerous reporters and private individuals over the course of several decades; it has been widely repeated in popular magazines, books, and contemporary newspapers. For the most complete telling during his lifetime, see A. J. Liebling, "Patron of the Preemies," *The New Yorker*, June 3, 1939, pp. 20–24.

18 **William Randolph Hearst had a genius idea:** Ibid.; see also William A. Silverman, "Incubator-Baby Side Shows," *Pediatrics* 64, no. 2 (August 1979), p. 137. Silverman notes that Chicago nurse Evelyn Lundeen told him that Couney was convinced all the quintuplets would die. I speculate that he also didn't want his secret to slip out: Martin Couney always had physicians on his payroll, which would have been hard to finesse in rural Canada. Finally, there's the possibility that the decision wasn't his: the *Tribune* reported that the Canadian obstetrician opposed a plan that would have moved the quintuplets to Chicago. "Doctor Vetoes Plans to Show 'Quints' at Fair," *Chicago Tribune*, May 31, 1934, p. 1.

19 **"We bring you the world's first Homecoming":** Infant incubator homecoming script for July 25, 1934, Century of Progress International Exposition Scrapbook.

19 **"All the world loves a baby":** Ibid.

The Obit That Wouldn't Die

20 **its plastic dome modeled on the B-29 bomber:** This information was provided to me by Dr. Lawrence Gartner, professor emeritus of pediatrics and obstetrics and gynecology at the University of Chicago and former chairman of the board of the American Pediatric Society, July 20, 1915.

20 **One theory held that since two- and three-pound humans:** William A. Silverman, *Retrolental Fibroplasia: A Modern Parable* (New York: Grune & Stratton, 1980), p. 76.

21 **If oxygen helped preemies breathe:** William A. Silverman, *Where's the Evidence? Debates in Modern Medicine* (New York: Oxford University Press, 1998), p. 2; Silverman, *Retrolental Fibroplasia.*

21 **No day was complete . . . he picked up the paper and saw:** William A. Silverman, address to colleagues at annual Newborn Dinner, April 30, 1970, recorded by Lawrence Gartner, M.D.

21 **Martin A. Couney, age eighty:** "Martin A. Couney, 'Incubator Doctor,'" *The New York Times*, March 2, 1950, p. 27.

22 **rare gigot:** Couney had a taste for rare gigot. A. J. Liebling, "Patron of the Preemies," *The New Yorker*, June 3, 1939, p. 21.

22 **at the mention of his late wife:** Jo Ranson, a Brooklyn reporter who frequently covered Couney during his lifetime, wrote that after Maye's death, he could

never mention her name without tears. Oliver Pilat and Jo Ranson, *Sodom by the Sea: An Affectionate History of Coney Island* (Garden City, NY: Doubleday, Doran, 1941), p. 194.

A Showman Is Born

23 **trouble rumbled across the border:** The Cohns were probably aware of the coming conflict. "War between France and Prussia was widely foreseen . . . in 1866," writes Michael Howard in *The Franco-Prussian War* (1961; London: Granada, 1979), p. 40. In 1939, Martin Couney told A. J. Liebling of *The New Yorker* that his family moved shortly *after* the Franco-Prussian War, but family records and vital statistics records indicate otherwise.

23 **Fredericke already had three children . . . this child would be her last:** It seems somehow fitting that Jewish birth records for that year and place do not exist, but I thank Anna Przybyszewska Drozd of the Jewish Genealogy & Family Heritage Center of the Emanuel Ringelblum Jewish Historical Institute in Warsaw for her endeavors on my behalf. Family information was compiled from numerous records, including Martin Couney's New York City marriage license, dated September 12, 1903; his passport application, dated November 8, 1904; and Alfons's burial certificate, dated February 6, 1949. In addition, information was provided to William Silverman by Martin Couney's niece, Ilsa, and her husband, Alfred Ephraim, most likely in the late 1960s. Lawrence Gartner gleaned more in 1980.

23 **Fredericke's people, the Levys, were doctors:** Silverman and Gartner, from the sources detailed in the previous note; reiterated by Ruth Freudenthal, Ilse Ephraim's daughter, interview with the author, August 18, 2015; it was Freudenthal who mentioned Napoleon.

23 **It was home to a well-known publisher:** Monasch Bar Loebel, *Lebenserinnerungen/Memoirs/Pamiętnik*. English trans. Peter Fraenkel, including a brief history of Krotoschin (Krotoszyn, Poland: Society of the Friends and Researchers of the Krotoszyn Region, 2004), pp. 83–98.

24 **If one saves a single life:** Sanhedrin 4:5.

24 **They were merchants:** Michael Simonson, archivist at the Leo Baeck Institute in New York, in correspondence with the author on October 20, 2015, provided the insight that many of the Jews in Krotoschin were secularized merchants and business owners, and that they left in search of opportunity and advancement.

24 **Only seventeen Jewish people:** "Krotoszyn," *The Encyclopedia of Jewish Life Before and During the Holocaust*, ed. Shmuel Spector and Geoffrey Wigoder (New York: New York University Press, 2001), vol. 2, p. 681. This article chronicles Krotoschin's population decline from the end of the nineteenth century through 1939.

Et Voilà! The Artificial Hen

25 **Not since Napoleon III walked these grounds:** For a description of this fair, including a comparison of the previous fair, in which "the proudest monarch upon earth moved before our view," see Henry Morford, *Paris and Half-Europe in '78: The Paris*

Exposition of 1878, Its Side-Shows and Excursions (New York: Geo. W. Carleton and Morford's Travel Publication Office, 1879), p. 6.

25 **The purpose was to show the world that France was back:** Ibid., p. 17.

26 **The literal French birth rate:** Jeffrey P. Baker, *The Machine in the Nursery: Incubator Technology and the Origins of Newborn Care* (Baltimore: Johns Hopkins University Press, 1996), p. 45.

26 **Dr. Étienne Tarnier was passing the afternoon:** Ibid., p. 26.

26 **This population plunge was deeply troubling:** Alisa Klaus, *Every Child a Lion: The Origins of Maternal and Infant Health Policy in the United States and France, 1890–1920* (Ithaca, NY: Cornell University Press, 1993), pp. 14–15.

26 **Tarnier had developed axis-traction forceps:** Walter Radcliffe, *Milestones in Midwifery and the Secret Instrument* (San Francisco: Norman Publishing, 1989), p. 93.

26 **Under 2,000 grams (4.4 pounds), maybe seven months' gestation:** Jeffrey P. Baker, "The Incubator Controversy: Pediatricians and the Origins of Premature Infant Technology in the United States, 1890 to 1910," *Pediatrics* 87, no. 5 (May 1991), p. 655; Baker, *The Machine in the Nursery*, p. 21.

26 **The Jardin d'Acclimatation:** The history of the zoo, including the eating of animals, and the human zoo, can be found on the Jardin d'Acclimatation website: http://jardindacclimatation.fr/150-ans-dhistoire/. Castor and Pollux have disappeared from that site but are discussed in numerous other sources, including Richard D. E. Burton, *Blood in the City: Violence and Revelation in Paris, 1789–1945* (Ithaca, NY: Cornell University Press, 2001), p. 319.

27 **the new machines designed for hatching and fattening:** *Guide du promeneur au Jardin Zoologique d'Acclimatation* (Paris: Jardin Zoologique d'Acclimatation du Bois de Boulogne, March 1, 1878), p. 27.

27 **At Leipzig Maternity Hospital:** Baker, *The Machine in the Nursery*, pp. 28–30. It isn't entirely clear exactly when Credé began using the *Warmewänne*. Baker speculates that it was about twenty years before Tarnier's epiphany; other accounts figure at least ten. (The warming tub in St. Petersburg, Russia, preceded Credé; it's generally dated to 1835.) By all accounts, Credé was using a kind of incubation well ahead of Tarnier and, according to Baker, was irritated by his rival's claims. Further notice of Credé and his machine can be found in "The Use of Incubators for Infants," *The Lancet* 1 (May 29, 1897), pp. 1490–1491.

27 **Peasants would try to save their weakling babies:** Ibid.

28 **But Carl Credé's rival would publish first:** Baker, *The Machine in the Nursery*, p. 30.

28 **By 1880, Étienne Tarnier had his *couveuse*:** Ibid., pp. 27–28.

29 **Tarnier reported that his *couveuse* cut the mortality rate:** Ibid.

29 **stewing the patients . . . To skirt that gruesome risk:** Ibid.

29 **Pierre Budin . . . must have had it in his mind:** Ibid., p. 49, notes that Auvard's star subsequently sank while Budin's rose.

William Silverman and the Couney Buffs Convene

30 **Illinois Nurse of the Year:** Two clippings from unidentified Chicago newspapers: Lois Wille, "Saving Premature Babies Her Job for 34 Years" (probably *Chicago Daily News*), October 14, 1958, and Nancy McGill, "Illinois Nurse of the Year," October 17,

1958, both in Julius Hays Hess Papers, Box 1, Folder 13, Special Collections Research Center, University of Chicago Library.

30 **During an afternoon spent feeding martinis:** William A. Silverman, address to colleagues at annual Newborn Dinner, April 30, 1970, recorded by Lawrence Gartner, M.D.; William A. Silverman, "Incubator-Baby Side Shows," *Pediatrics* 64, no. 2 (August 1979), p. 137.

31 **Drs. Silverman, Gartner, and Butterfield began to call themselves:** Lawrence Gartner, interview with the author, July 20, 2015.

31 **people strained to capture fraying threads of memory:** This is my assessment, based on listening to numerous tape recordings of interviews conducted by Lawrence and Carol Gartner.

31 **"He wasn't pretentious, he was real nice to you":** Jerome Champion, interview with Lawrence Gartner, April 1970.

31 **"I've always felt a little bit concerned":** Silverman, address at 1970 Newborn Dinner, recorded by Gartner.

Michael Cohn Sees an Elephant, and the Light of a New World

33 **hopeful and wistful and nervy with fear:** Martin Couney did not leave any impressions of his emigration, which was more than ten years earlier than he wanted everyone to believe. For a depiction of the journey to port and the trip across the Atlantic, I relied on archival letters from German immigrants who made the crossing in the same time period, in Walter D. Kamphoefner, Wolfgang Helbich, and Ulrike Sommer, eds., *News from the Land of Freedom: German Immigrants Write Home*, trans. Susan Carter Vogel (Ithaca, NY: Cornell University Press, 1993).

34 **at the port of Hamburg, an eighteen-year-old:** The ship manifest of the *Gellert* (Manifest ID 00040642; National Archives identifier 1746067) and the arrival records at Castle Garden (Castlegarden.org), the immigrant intake center that preceded Ellis Island, confirm the passage of eighteen-year-old "Martin" Cohn from Krotoschin, steerage class. (This jibes with later records, such as his naturalization and his passport application, where he refers to his 1888 arrival.) It's possible that he was already using the name Martin rather than Michael at the time of boarding.

35 **His father had died:** A death record for Hermann Cohn has not been found. William A. Silverman, "Incubator-Baby Side Shows," *Pediatrics* 64, no. 2 (August 1979), p. 127, says that Martin's father died when he was young. This information was most likely provided to Silverman by Ilsa Ephraim, Martin Couney's niece.

35 **His brother Alfons emigrated first:** Fifteen-year-old Alfons Hugo Cohn arrived at Castle Garden on November 8, 1882. Castlegarden.org.

35 **Jaunty, stylish Alfons:** Alfons is described as a "stylish Frenchman" in an account of his 1893 arrest over a fight at the Gravesend (Coney Island) racetrack, "A Story of Assault," *The Brooklyn Daily Eagle*, September 12, 1893, p. 5. William Silverman, most likely drawing from his conversation with Ilse Ephraim, noted that Alfons was a jockey. Alfons's March 29, 1894, naturalization in New York County's Superior Court lists his occupation as "clerk." A New York newspaper article about "missing persons," titled "Anybody Seen These?" (*The World*, June 3, 1896, p. 4), states that "former [New York City] Register Ferdinand Levy received a very pathetic letter a few days ago from Fredericka [sic] Cohn of Krotochin." She was searching for her son Alfons, who had left home about fifteen years before and had been a bank clerk; he also had racehorses.

35 **The pachyderm-shaped building was the Elephant Hotel:** Coney Island lore holds that immigrants' first sight of the New World during this time was the bizarre Elephant Colossus. This was explained to me by Jay Singer, a docent at the Coney Island Museum. An excellent description of the hotel can be found in Edo McCullough, *Good Old Coney Island: A Sentimental Journey into the Past* (1957; New York: Fordham University Press, 2000), p. 55; another, stating that it was the first edifice seen by immigrants, is in Michael Immerso, *Coney Island: The People's Playground* (New Brunswick, NJ: Rutgers University Press, 2002), p. 38.

The Couney Buffs Encounter the Mysterious M. Lion

36 **"colorful (and bizarre!) chapter in medical history":** William A. Silverman, "Incubator-Baby Side Shows," *Pediatrics* 64, no. 2 (August 1979), p. 127.
36 **"whether neonatal medicine's enormous increase":** William A. Silverman, *Where's the Evidence? Debates in Modern Medicine* (New York: Oxford University Press, 1998), p. 4. The book is a compilation of Silverman's previous essays over the decades.
38 **a credible-sounding reader named Felix Marx:** William A. Silverman, "Postscript to Incubator-Baby Side Shows," *Pediatrics* 66, no. 3 (September 1980), pp. 474–475 (letters).

"The Greatest Novelty of the Age!"

39 **born in Kraków:** Most of Samuel Schenkein's paperwork cites Kraków. To travel from New York to London in 1897 did not require a passport. Interestingly, in his 1900 passport application (no. 20343), Schenkein stated his birthplace as Brooklyn. However, he also declared his profession as "merchant," then crossed that out and wrote "retired"—which was most certainly not the case. This document was witnessed by M. A. Couney. Couney later declared himself "retired" in his 1904 passport application (no. 95148). I suspect "retired" was a way of avoiding questions and/or tariffs.
39 **More than one hundred thousand . . . Six thousand women:** James Walter Smith, "Baby Incubators," *The Strand Magazine* (London) 12 (July–December 1896), p. 776.
39 **had secured exclusive rights for London for this summer:** See the letter signed by Schenkein and Coney, later in this chapter. A photo published in the London *Times* clearly shows the machines are licensed from German instrument maker Paul Altmann. The paper, in an untitled item, also mentions Altmann's patent: *The Times*, July 15, 1897, p. 3. Next in the listings is the Royal Aquarium, which had not yet acquired its own preemies.
40 **Every day, with something like 3,600 people:** "The Danger of Making a Public Show of Incubators for Babies," *The Lancet* 1 (February 5, 1898), p. 390.
40 **The spiel might go like this:** This is based on Couney's later documented interactions with the crowds, and his incessant courting of physicians.
40 **"The employment of incubators as a means" . . . "The main feature of this new incubator":** "The Use of Incubators for Infants," *The Lancet* 1 (May 29, 1897), pp. 1490–1491.
40 **the feeding . . . and the cleaning:** Ibid. A similar description is found in "To Teach the Young Idea How to Shoot," *The Sketch: A Journal of Art and Actuality,* August 24,

1897, p. 195. An accompanying photograph shows "Paul Altmann Patents" in large letters on the wall.

41 **awkward, wheeled brooder:** This machine is described in Jeffrey P. Baker, *The Machine in the Nursery: Incubator Technology and the Origins of Newborn Intensive Care* (Baltimore: Johns Hopkins University Press, 1996), p. 71. Rotch partnered with a technical expert named John Pickering Putnam, but the thing was clunky and short-lived.

41 **the superior system that he, Alexandre Lion, devised:** Smith, "Baby Incubators," pp. 770–776.

42 **"just big enough" . . . "like the bearded lady":** Ibid., pp. 770, 772.

43 **the only person not convinced was Dr. Pierre Budin:** Pierre Budin, *The Nursling*, trans. William J. Maloney (London: Caxton, 1907), Lecture 1, p. 13.

43 **At Maternité, the rudimentary *couveuse*:** "It is far better to put the little one in an incubator by its mother's bedside," Budin said. Baker, *The Machine in the Nursery*, p. 150.

43 **Breast, breast, breast:** Ibid., pp. 49–55.

43 **he also used *gavage*:** Budin, *The Nursling*, Lecture 2, p. 28.

44 **Alexandre Lion was strategic:** In the 1990s, Drs. Lawrence Gartner and L. Joseph Butterfield enlisted two German physicians to help with reconnaissance missions. Leonore Ballowitz, M.D., discovered a sketch of a *Kinderbrutanstalt* published in the 1896 issue of *Berliner Ilustrirte Zeitung*, and other documentation supporting that the exhibit was the work of Lion. The second researcher, Julia Whitefield, M.D., Ph.D., who'd moved from Frankfurt to Arvada, Colorado, translated the "Official Exhibition News" from 1896. This document spoke of Rudolf Virchow's approval, the Germans' desire to make the exhibition permanent, and Lion's declining the offer, while volunteering to donate the machines. (The document is cited in "Martin Couney's Story Revisited," letter to the editor, *Pediatrics* 100, no. 1 [July 1997], p. 159.) Both women also saw Lion's *Patentschrift*. Correspondence belonging to Lawrence Gartner shows that for a time, the buffs speculated that Martin Couney might have been Lion's assistant. Searching archives in the former East Berlin, Dr. Ballowitz learned that Lion did have an assistant—but that man's name was Leotardi. In a final effort at extending the benefit of the doubt to Martin Couney, some of the buffs wondered if Lion and Couney were actually the same person. Subsequent discoveries, including Couney's immigration papers and photographs of the two men, put that theory soundly to bed.

44 **His clients included Robert Koch:** Lawrence M. Gartner and Carol B. Gartner, "The Care of Premature Infants: Historical Perspective," in *Neonatal Intensive Care: A History of Excellence*, A Symposium Commemorating Child Health Day, NIH Publication No. 92-2786 (Bethesda, MD: National Institutes of Health, 1992), http://www.neonatology.org/classics/nic.nih1985.pdf. See also Baker, *The Machine in the Nursery*, p. 95.

44 **"Little children have ever been esteemed":** "Immature Infants in France," *The Lancet* 1 (January 16, 1897), p. 196.

44 **"The Greatest Novelty of the Age!":** Unidentified newspaper clipping, 1897, provided to me by Dr. Lawrence Gartner. The name of the publication is missing, but the item appears to be a paid listing.

44 **"It works automatically":** "To Teach the Young Idea How to Shoot," p. 195.

45 **Just get your own and say it was smaller:** In his 1905 account of treating babies at the St. Louis World's Fair, Dr. John Zahorsky notes an 1898 editorial in *Pediatrics*, reporting that Barnum & Bailey had a twenty-ounce baby ("Incubators in London,"

Pediatrics 5 [April 1, 1898], pp. 298–299); Zahorsky speculated that this "data" came from an English newspaper. John Zahorsky, *Baby Incubators: A Clinical Study of the Premature Infant, with Especial Reference to Incubator Institutions Conducted for Show Purposes* (St. Louis: Courier of Medicine, 1905), p. 12. Barring a miracle, that weight seems impossibly low for that time.

45 **"Sirs, In the interests of the general public":** Samuel Schenkein and Martin Coney, "Infant Incubators," letter to the editor, *The Lancet* 2 (September 18, 1897), p. 744. Although the top signature is Schenkein's, it is my belief that the letter was written by "Coney." I have found no other documents written by Mr. Schenkein, but I have found many letters composed by Martin Couney, and this one matches his style.

46 **While the "favourably noticed" exhibit:** "The Danger of Making a Public Show of Incubators for Babies," *The Lancet* 1 (February 5, 1898), pp. 390–391.

47 **Already he'd spent a night in jail:** "A Story of Assault," *The Brooklyn Daily Eagle,* September 12, 1893, p. 5.

The March of Science and Industry

51 **"Individuals, groups, entire races of man fall into step":** *Official Guide Book of the Fair, 1933* (Chicago: A Century of Progress, 1933), p. 11.

53 **"I loved Coney Island like a person":** Paul Brigandi, Coney Island memorabilia collector, interview with the author, June 15, 2015.

The Arrival of the Eminent Dr. Martin Arthur Couney

55 **The gangly man had a hatbox in his hands:** Martin Couney related the story of the hatbox baby in A. J. Liebling, "Patron of the Preemies," *The New Yorker,* June 3, 1939, p. 23. This anecdote and Couney's Chicago show inspired the novel *The Hatbox Baby* by Carrie Brown (Chapel Hill, NC: Algonquin Books, 2000).

56 **The original White City . . . had set a new American standard:** For the best depiction of the White City and its significance, see Erik Larson, *The Devil in the White City: Murder, Magic, and Madness at the Fair That Changed America* (New York: Crown, 2003).

57 **No "spirituous liquors" sold:** James B. Hayes, *History of the Trans-Mississippi and International Exhibition of 1898* (St. Louis: Woodward & Tiernan, 1910), p. 51, http://trans-mississippi.unl.edu/texts/view/transmiss.book.haynes.1910.html.

57 **"To the spectator it would seem that some long forgotten magician":** *The Omaha Bee,* front-page story on the fair's opening day (June 1, 1898), cited in the Trans-Mississippi and International Exposition digital archive, University of Nebraska–Lincoln, http://trans-mississippi.unl.edu/.

57 **the "savages" . . . "The gay throngs":** John A. Wakefield, *A History of the Trans-Mississippi International Exposition* (May 1903), http://trans-mississippi.unl.edu/texts/view/transmiss.book.wakefield.1903.html.

57 **"WONDERFUL INVENTION" and "Visited by 207,000 People at Queen Victoria's Diamond Jubilee":** F. A. Rinehart photograph, F. A. Rinehart Collection, Omaha Public Library.

57 **Reporters ignored him:** Press reports of the incubator station appear to be nonexistent. L. Joseph Butterfield, "The Incubator Doctor in Denver: A Medical Missing

Link," in *The 1970 Denver Westerners Brand Book*, ed. Jackson C. Thode (Denver: Denver Westerners, 1971), p. 350, writes that "a careful search of 12 heavy volumes of clippings about the Exposition has failed to reveal a single reference."

57 **The infants on display might not have been as tiny:** The babies and their care remain a bit of a mystery. In 1939, Couney told A. J. Liebling of *The New Yorker* that he'd brought them from Chicago—a feat that seems highly improbable, unless these little ones were not really so little. With neither Louise Recht nor Maye Segner on hand, it's not clear who was nursing them. In "The Incubator Doctor in Denver," p. 350, L. Joseph Butterfield mentioned correspondence with Dr. Warren Bosley of Grand Island, Nebraska; the latter reported that a woman who'd visited the Omaha exposition several times when she was eleven didn't recall seeing any nurses, nor did she see the babies taken out of the machines.

58 **the naked French painting:** Hayes, *History of the Trans-Mississippi and International Exposition of 1898*, p. 207.

58 **The show he opened at 2 West Eighteenth Street:** Cited in numerous newspaper articles, among them "The Lion Institute Opened," *New-York Tribune*, October 26, 1897, p. 9; see also *American Medico-Surgical Bulletin* 11 (November 10, 1897), p. 1002. The articles say that Lion would leave the station in the hands of a New York physician. After that, mention of it in any popular or medical publications ends. Given that the Buffalo show in 1901 made a tremendous splash as a unique endeavor, I have concluded the Manhattan station was gone by then. Lion left so light a footprint in New York that the Couney buffs were not even aware he had ever set up shop.

58 **"Dr. Martin Couney says nursing mothers":** These ads appeared throughout October and November 1898 in the *Omaha World-Herald* and *The Nebraska State Journal*, including October 27 and 30 and November 4, 9, 10, 14, 15, 16, and 23. The one specifically stating "a wide experience" appeared in the *Omaha World-Herald*, October 27, p. 8, and in *The Omaha Daily Bee*, October 30, part II, p. 13.

59 **Martin A. *Coney* was an American citizen:** The index card on file at the National Archives (Certificate of Naturalization vol. C-2, p. 15, Jour. vol. 59, p. 503) is typewritten as "Coney." Martin's original signed document on file at the Nebraska State Historical Society (vol. C-2, p. 14, of the journal cited above) shows his signature with an accent *aigu* over the *e*.

Nailing Jelly to the Wall: The Couney Buffs Gain a Follower

60 **"We write this letter to your readers":** "Martin Couney's Story Revisited," letter to the editor, *Pediatrics* 100, no. 1 (July 1997), pp. 159–160.

60 **His *New York Times* obituary:** Jennifer Bayot, "William A. Silverman, 87, Dies; Leading Neonatologist of 1950's," *The New York Times*, January 2, 2005, http://www.nytimes.com/2005/01/02/nyregion/william-a-silverman-87-dies-leading-neonatologist-of-1950s.html.

"The President Has Been Shot!"

61 **another Paris Universelle Exposition:** Erik Mattie, *World's Fairs* (New York: Princeton Architectural Press, 1998), p. 101.

61 **M. Lion printed copious souvenir postcards:** I had no trouble finding one on eBay in 2015.

61 **Martin Coney signed a business agreement with Samuel Schenkein:** The date and details of their agreement emerged in the company's subsequent bankruptcy proceedings; see *In re Schenkein et al.* (District Court, Western District New York, February 7, 1902), No. 763, *The Federal Reporter*, vol. 113, pp. 421–429. Newspapers at the time refer to McConnell as Emmett H., while legal documents refer to Emmett W.

61 *Cue-BAY-tah:* The perspicacious William Silverman picked up on the name Qbata as an "echo-nym." William A. Silverman, "Incubator-Baby Side Shows," *Pediatrics* 64, no. 2 (August 1979), p. 127.

61 **The Kny-Scheerer company in New York manufactured:** T. E. Cone, *History of the Care and Feeding of the Premature Infant* (Boston: Little, Brown, 1985), p. 55.

62 **Chicago Lying-in:** Joseph Bolivar DeLee, "Chicago Lying-in Hospital and Dispensary," Northwestern Medical School Yearbook, 1903, clipping from the collection of Dr. Lawrence Gartner.

62 **Low Maternity in Brooklyn:** Frances H. Stuart, "De Lion Incubator at Low Maternity Hospital," *Brooklyn Medical Journal* 15 (1901), pp. 346–349.

62 **Sloane Maternity:** James D. Voorhees, "The Care of Premature Babies in Incubators," *Archives of Pediatrics* 17 (1900), pp. 331–346, discusses the care of preemies at Sloane, where he was a resident physician. He describes the Lion model as the best available but notes that the hospital was so strapped for resources that sometimes three babies were placed in one machine, and sometimes babies were removed early because of demand. In addition to the Lion machines, the hospital used cheap modifications of the Tarnier or Auvard *couveuse.*

62 **Copycat contraptions:** Jeffrey P. Baker, "The Incubator Controversy: Pediatricians and the Origins of Premature Infant Technology in the United States, 1890 to 1910," *Pediatrics* 87, no. 5 (May 1991), pp. 655–656; for one example of a homemade warming crib, see John Bartlett, "The Warming-Crib," *The Chicago Medical Journal and Examiner* 54 (May 1887), pp. 449–454.

62 **First on the agenda:** *In re Schenkein et al.,* pp. 421–429.

63 **Sam found an investor, Emmett W. McConnell:** Ibid.

63 **"Dr. Coney":** Martin Couney is called Dr. Coney in every newspaper and magazine article I could find about this show, and there were many.

63 **Miss Annabelle Maye Segner:** "Wife of Nationally Known Physician Worked with Mate for Many Years," obituary, *The Brooklyn Daily Eagle*, February 23, 1936.

63 **the favorite child:** Annabelle Maye Segner's widowed mother lived with the couple from the time of their marriage until her death; she left almost all of her money to Maye.

64 **she gave it a bath in "synized" water and mustard:** "Tiny Mites of Humanity Receive Most Assiduous Care from Nurses and Physicians," *Buffalo Express*, June 12, 1901.

65 **Every two hours, those who could suckle were carried upstairs:** "Baby Incubators at the Pan-American Exposition," *Scientific American* 85, no. 5 (August 3, 1901), p. 68.

65 **free season passes from Sam, signed "Dr. Schenkein":** I have seen microfiche of the one that was given to Dr. Matthew D. Mann. Buffalo History Museum Research Library, M82-5, Dr. Matthew D. Mann Scrapbooks.

65 **Little Willie . . . the twin girls . . . The baby boy, A.S.:** "Tiny Mites of Humanity Receive Most Assiduous Care from Nurses and Physicians."

Notes

66 **triplets arrived:** "Marked the Triplets for Identification: And Then They Were Placed in an Incubator—Watched by Mother," *Saginaw Evening News* (Michigan; dateline Buffalo), July 22, 1901.

66 **Yet his eyes, in the moment when the shutter was released:** Photograph (figure 6) in William A. Silverman, "Incubator-Baby Side Shows," *Pediatrics* 64, no. 2 (August 1979), p. 133.

66 *The Buffalo News* **declared "it":** *The Buffalo News*, July 20, 1901, as cited at http://library.buffalo.edu/pan-am/exposition/health/medical/incubators.html.

66 *Pediatrics* **judged the exhibit instructive:** "Exhibit of Infant Incubators at the Pan-American Exposition," *Pediatrics* 12 (1901), pp. 414–419.

66 *Scientific American* **repeated the 85 percent survival rate:** "Baby Incubators at the Pan-American Exposition," p. 68.

66 **waxing ecstatic in the pages of** *Cosmopolitan:* Arthur Brisbane, "The Incubator Baby and Niagara Falls," *Cosmopolitan* 31 (September 1901), pp. 509–516.

67 **"The question naturally presents itself":** "Some Medical Aspects of the Pan American Exposition: Infant Incubators," *Buffalo Medical Journal* 57, no. 1 (August 1901; reprinted from *Boston Medical and Surgical Journal*, July 18, 1901), p. 56.

68 **he was someone for whom the term "pillar of society":** The depiction of Dr. Mann, and description of his club activities, complimentary season passes, and presence on the opening day of the fair, are drawn from the Dr. Matthew D. Mann Scrapbooks, Buffalo History Museum Research Library, M82-5.

68 **Colleagues of his apparently were sending their patients:** Local doctors were sending their patients to the concession, and the well-connected Dr. Mann would almost certainly have been acquainted with some of them. The *Buffalo Medical Journal* 57, no. 1 (August 1901), noted one arrival from a prominent family. Whether Dr. Mann sent any of his own patients is unknown.

69 **A former architecture student from Irontown, Ohio:** The partnership of Thompson and Dundy is chronicled in Oliver Pilat and Jo Ranson, *Sodom by the Sea: An Affectionate History of Coney Island* (Garden City, NY: Doubleday, Doran, 1941), pp. 142–143. I have seen other versions of the details of this story (as often happens with Coney Island lore), but all agree they were rivals in Omaha and became partners in Buffalo in 1901. Pilat and Ranson's version is the most common.

69 **"The visitor witnesses the punishment meted out to scandal-mongers":** *Official Catalogue and Guide Book to the Pan-American Exhibition*, May 1–November 1, 1901 (Buffalo: Charles Ahrhart, 1901), p. 45.

70 **one Edward M. Bayliss of St. Louis:** The showman's biography and previous extravaganzas are presented in *World's Fair Bulletin*, Published in the Interest of the Louisiana Purchase Exposition (St. Louis: World's Fair Publishing Company, March 1902), p. 36.

70 **"Expositions are the timekeepers of progress":** This quotation is widely cited. For one source, see "President McKinley's Last Public Utterance to the People in Buffalo, New York," September 5, 1901, Gerhard Peters and John T. Woolley, *The American Presidency Project*, http://www.presidency.ucsb.edu/ws/?pid=69326.

71 **That evening, McKinley and his wife, unaware of the near-assassination:** Captioned images of the president's two days at the fair can be found at the University at Buffalo (State University of New York) Libraries' online collection: Pan-American Exposition of 1901, "Images of President William McKinley at the Pan-American Exposition," http://library.buffalo.edu/pan-am/exposition/law/mckinley.html.

71 **George B. Courtelyou, thought it a bad idea:** A. Wesley Johns, *The Man Who Shot McKinley* (South Brunswick, NJ: A. S. Barnes, 1970), p. 20.

71 **three thousand inside and another ten thousand outside:** Among other sources, this appears in a newspaper clipping from the New York *Sun*, September 7, 1901, kept in the scrapbook of the surgeon Matthew Mann, Buffalo History Museum Research Library, M82-5, Dr. Matthew D. Mann Scrapbooks.

71 **"Be easy with him, boys":** Among other popular sources, "The Assassination of President William McKinley, 1901," Eyewitness to History, www.eyewitnessto history.com/mckinley.htm. It is also relayed as "Let no one hurt him"; see Marshall Everett, *Complete Life of William McKinley and Story of His Assassination: An Authentic and Official Memorial Edition* . . . (Chicago: C. W. Stanton, 1901), p. 36; and Nelson W. Wilson, "Details of President McKinley's Case," *Buffalo Medical Journal* 57, no. 3 (October 1901), p. 207. Another account, "Official Report of the Assassination," *The New York Times*, September 14, 1901, describes the assassin being pinned but makes no mention of any such words.

71 **the ambulance had to pass directly in front:** A map of the exposition shows the only possible route from the Temple of Music; the medical center and the incubator exhibition were so close that one account described them as being next door to each other.

72 **Martin, so close yet so bereft of credentials:** Years later, Couney would tell his niece and her husband about his proximity to the emergency medical center, without mentioning his lack of credentials: Ilsa Ephraim, interview with Lawrence Gartner, January 4, 1980.

72 **Inside the medical center, as Buffalo's physicians:** Wilson, "Details of President McKinley's Case," pp. 208–215.

72 **"the blood of the Republic":** Ibid., p. 210.

72 **Dr. Mann had five other doctors:** Ibid., pp. 210–215.

72 **the first Nobel Prize in Physics:** Nobelprize.org, https://www.nobelprize.org/nobel_prizes/themes/physics/karlsson/index.html.

72 **Dr. Park arrived just as the operation was ending:** Wilson, "Details of President McKinley's Case," p. 214. It's unclear who did the actual stitching.

72 **At first, McKinley seemed to rally:** Dr. Mann, clearly shaken, kept copies of daily press updates in his scrapbooks. The initial optimism was also recorded in Wilson, "Details of President McKinley's Case," pp. 215–216.

73 **"It's God's way":** McKinley's last words were widely reported on the front page of newspapers throughout the country with a few words' variation. In some versions, he also quotes from the hymn "Nearer, My God, to Thee."

73 **"BABIES MAY DIE":** "Babies May Die," *Jackson Citizen Patriot* (Michigan), November 11, 1901, p. 1. *In re Schenkein et al.* implies that both Schenkein and Coney were arrested, but newspapers at the time report only Schenkein's. Had the popular "Dr. Coney" been detained as well, I believe, the press would have been on it.

73 **Deputy Sheriff Michael Burke was babysitting:** "Baby Incubators Seized by Sheriff," *The Charlotte Observer*, November 12, 1901, p. 7.

73 **a judge would vacate the order of arrest:** Newspaper articles state that it occurred the same day as the arrest, although a ledger held in the National Archives indicates February 3: "In the matter of the petition Samuel Schenkein & Martin Couney, indiv and as co partners," recorded in United States District Court, Western District of New York, document 763, stamped June 30, 1903.

73 **They were sent home:** "Baby Incubators Seized by Sheriff," p. 7.

74 **Children's Hospital bought a few machines:** Baker, *The Machine in the Nursery: Incubator Technology and the Origins of Newborn Intensive Care* (Baltimore: Johns Hopkins University Press, 1996), p. 99.

Welcome to the City of the Dead

75 **Proceed along a long and curving road:** I visited Cypress Hills Cemetery in Brooklyn on April 15, 2015.
76 **Kirschenbaum's Westminster Chapel:** "Dr. Martin A. Couney Dies; Incubator Baby Pioneer," *The Brooklyn Daily Eagle*, March 2, 1950, p. 19.
77 **"Re: Martin Couney, M.D.":** Letter from Harold S. Musselwhite, Jr., to Research Librarian, June 27, 1996, Newborn Medicine History Collection, Pediatric History Center, American Academy of Pediatrics.
77 **"My parents and several others were preparing":** Letter from Harold S. Musselwhite, Jr., to L. Joseph Butterfield, M.D., June 6, 1996, Newborn Medicine History Collection, Pediatric History Center, American Academy of Pediatrics.
77 **obituary for Harold Musselwhite, Jr.:** *The Berkshire Eagle*, February 27, 2005, via Legacy.com, http://www.legacy.com/obituaries/berkshire/obituary.aspx?n=harold-musselwhite&pid=3220428.
78 **The "incubator twins" from the Century of Progress:** Jami Kunzer, "'Incubator Twins': Once on Display as 'Living Babies,' Sisters Celebrate 80th Birthdays," *Northwest Herald* (Crystal Lake, Illinois), August 23, 2014, http://www.nwherald.com/2014/08/21/incubator-twins-once-on-display-as-living-babies-sisters-celebrate-80th-birthdays/anleac5/.
78 **Jane had the flat midwestern accent of my childhood:** Jane Umbarger, interview with the author, November 10, 2014.
79 **both women on the line:** Jane Umbarger and Jean Harrison, interview with the author, November 5, 2015.

Two Elephants, a Wedding, and a Bunch of Crying Babies

82 **a crowd of invited guests gathered to witness a public execution:** Alas, there are more versions of this story than Topsy had legs. Some claim it was the doing of Thomas Edison, trying to win the "current wars," but most insist that Edison supplied only the electricity, while Thompson and Dundy supplied the motive. Front-page newspaper stories at the time bear out that theory. "Wicked Topsy Must Die," read a headline in the New York *Sun* on January 3, 1903, and then, "Kill Topsy Humanely—Thompson & Dundy Must Not Make a Sideshow of Her Death." I compiled this account from several sources, most heavily "Coney Island Elephant Killed," *The New York Times*, January 3, 1903, p. 1, and "Poisoned and Electrocuted," *Democrat and Chronicle* (Rochester, New York), January 5, 1903, p. 1.
83 **Samuel Schenkein was back from the brink:** *In re Schenkein et al.* (District Court, Western District New York, February 7, 1902), No. 763, *The Federal Reporter*, vol. 113, pp. 421–429, details the legal arguments put forth, while dates of motions and discharge are held by the National Archives, in "In the matter of the petition Samuel Schenkein & Martin Couney, indiv and as co partners," recorded in United States District Court, Western District of New York, document 763, stamped June 30, 1903. The "petitioner" received payment, but the amount was not recorded. Unfortunately, the complete records of the case were not retained, and parts of the handwritten ledger entries are illegible.
84 **On April 27, who should arrive aboard *La Gascogne*:** Ship manifest of *La Gascogne*, via Ellis Island Passenger Search (Passenger ID 102638030262). Louise Recht's

immediate destination was Schenkein's office. Tantalizingly, the manifest states she had been in the United States once before, but I can find no record of that earlier visit. In 1924, her certificate of naturalization (32431) would give her arrival as March 14, 1903; I suspect that was a lapse in memory.

84 **"Come this way, ladies and gentlemen!":** "Hints to Young Parents in Luna Park 'Qbators,'" *The Brooklyn Daily Eagle*, June 4, 1903, p. 3.

84 **The middle class unbuttoned:** A good description of Coney Island at this time is found in John F. Kasson, *Amusing the Million: Coney Island at the Turn of the Century* (New York: Hill and Wang, 1978), pp. 42–43.

85 **He drew up a cunning second-year contract:** For Tilyou's dealings with Thompson and Dundy, see Edo McCullough, *Good Old Coney Island: A Sentimental Journey into the Past* (1957; New York: Fordham University Press, 2000), pp. 302–303.

86 **"Strangest Place on Earth for Human Tots to Be Fed, Nursed and Cared For":** Subhead of "Hints to Young Parents in Luna Park 'Qbators.'"

86 **"haranguing the passing throng":** Ibid.

87 **Doubtless he'd have visited, if he hadn't been three thousand miles away:** Alfons made San Francisco news by suing the Market Street Railway Company for injuries sustained in December of 1900. "Street Railway Damage Suits," *San Francisco Chronicle*, March 1, 1901, p. 5. From everything I can gather, he remained in San Francisco for the rest of his life.

86 **he dared a fellow member of the San Francisco Olympic Club:** Barry Spitz, *Dipsea: The Greatest Race* (San Anselmo, CA: Potrero Meadow, 1993), p. 1. The race is still run every year.

87 **he and Annabelle Maye signed their marriage license:** New York City Marriage Bureau Records, certificate number 19262.

87 **On October 1, his change of name was finalized:** I found a copy of this signed documentation, with an official seal, on file with Hildegarde Couney's 1956 will, file 4847, at the Kings County Surrogate Court Archive. It is accompanied by a confirmation from the German consulate, numbered 7691.

Kiss the Baby

88 **The child was named Beth Bernstein:** Beth (Bernstein) Allen, interview with the author, October 25, 2014. All of Beth Allen's quotations in this chapter are from that interview.

91 **"A lot of people expressed horror":** Terry Silverman, undated interview with Elinoar Astrinsky for the Coney Island History Project, http://www.coneyislandhistory .org/oral-history-archive/terry-silverman.

91 **"She was the star of the show":** Ibid.

"The Crime of the Decade"

94 **Dreamland was intended as the lifted-pinkie answer:** Edo McCullough, *Good Old Coney Island: A Sentimental Journey into the Past* (1957; New York: Fordham University Press, 2000), pp. 192–196. The Coney Island Museum has an excellent trove of images.

94 **On August 1, he ripped a page from Alexandre Lion's playbook:** The event was widely publicized throughout the United States; one example is "Incubator Babies Hold a Reunion," *Tampa Tribune*, August 3, 1904 (dateline New York, August 2).

95 **"New York Excited over the Smallest Living Body":** The story of Baby Lillian ran in papers across the country. This headline was in the Milwaukee *Wisconsin Weekly Advocate*, August 11, 1904, p. 1.

95 **"The case of Lillian is, of course, the most wonderful":** Ibid.

95 **another in Minneapolis (for which he would "train" the personnel):** "The Incubator Babies at Wonderland Park," *The Minneapolis Journal*, May 20, 1905, p. 10; "Dr. Schenkein Tells of the Reasons for Exhibiting the Infant Incubators," *The Minneapolis Journal*, May 29, 1905, p. 4.

95 **Sam had been invited to make their pitch:** Minutes of the Committee on Concessions, October 3, 1901, Louisiana Purchase Exposition Company Records, Chouteau-Papin Collection, Missouri History Museum, St. Louis.

95 **they were shopping around:** Minutes of the Committee on Concessions, September 5, 1902.

96 **"I don't see why it is that you have any objection":** This entire conversation is from the Minutes of the Committee on Concessions, December 4, 1902. Published by permission of the Missouri History Museum, St. Louis.

98 **"a little difficulty":** Ibid.

98 ~~On January 22, 1903, Sam made another desperate pitch:~~ Minutes of the Committee on Concessions, January 22, 1903.

98 **Mrs. Hattie McCall Travis:** Untitled clipping from the Plainwell, Michigan, *News*, March 20, 1903, Louisiana Purchase Exposition Scrapbook, vol. 163, Chouteau-Papin Collection, Missouri History Museum, St. Louis. Her bid shows up in the committee's records as well; she was subsequently awarded a Spanish concession.

98 **Emmett McConnell himself:** Minutes of the Committee on Concessions, August 19, 1903.

98 **By August, Sam blinked:** Ibid.

98 **But Bayliss, the man with a hand inside:** Ibid.

98 **turn it over to Hardy:** Hardy (the partner cited in the World's Fair minutes) is also named as the physician in charge in the *World's Fair Bulletin*, April 1904, p. 20, Chouteau-Papin Collection, Missouri History Museum, St. Louis, as well as in numerous newspapers.

98 **Bayliss, to his credit, purchased Lion-type machines:** John Zahorsky, *Baby Incubators: A Clinical Study of the Premature Infant, with Especial Reference to Incubator Institutions Conducted for Show Purposes* (St. Louis: Courier of Medicine, 1905), p. 12.

98 **doctors were turning against them:** The precipitous decline of incubators in the early twentieth century is well summed up in Gerald Oppenheimer, "Prematurity as a Public Health Problem: US Policy from the 1920s to the 1960s," *American Journal of Public Health* 86, no. 6 (June 1996), pp. 870–878; also Jeffrey P. Baker, "The Incubator Controversy: Pediatricians and the Origins of Premature Infant Technology in the United States, 1890 to 1910," *Pediatrics* 87, no. 5 (May 1991).

100 **mothers and fathers started calling:** "Babies Sent to the Incubator from All Parts of the Country," *The St. Louis Republic*, July 17, 1904, p. 13; Zahorsky, *Baby Incubators*, pp. 38–39. It was Dr. Zahorsky who noted that most of those coming by train died en route.

100 **The first child to die had been sick:** Zahorsky, *Baby Incubators*, p. 29.

100 **Another baby followed, and another, and another:** The individual components of the debacle are detailed and sourced later in this chapter.

100 "I have never at any time had reason": Letter from A. N. Curtis, M.D., August 12, 1904, Executive Committee Minutes, Louisiana Purchase Exposition Company Records, Chouteau-Papin Collection, Missouri History Museum, St. Louis.

100 "serious objections . . . garbage boxes filled with filth": Letter from H. J. Scherck, M.D., August 11, 1904, Executive Committee Minutes.

100 "The feeding of the babies betrayed the grossest ignorance": Letter signed "City of St. Louis, Health Department," August 13, 1904, Executive Committee Minutes.

101 "Dear Sir, The Humane Society has been investigating": Letter from Rozier G. Meigs to David R. Francis, September 17, 1904, from the Louisiana Purchase Exposition Company Executive Committee Minutes, September 20, 1904. Published by permission of the Missouri History Museum, St. Louis.

102 "who is unable to take time" . . . "come as a complete surprise": Letter written on behalf of President Francis, September 19, 1904, from the Louisiana Purchase Exposition Company Executive Committee Minutes, September 20, 1904.

102 "It is horrible to think of these delicate babies": While this originally appeared in the *New York Evening Journal*, I was able to find it reprinted as "Incubators of Death," *The Denver Post*, September 15, 1904, p. 4.

102 "Dear Sir, The crime of the decade": Ibid.

104 Eager not only to save the day but also to win: Zahorsky had been rejected for membership in the elite American Pediatric Society in 1900 and experienced ongoing frustration, according to Jeffrey P. Baker, *The Machine in the Nursery: Incubator Technology and the Origins of Newborn Care* (Baltimore: Johns Hopkins University Press, 1996), p. 102.

104 pouring ice water into the coils of the machines: Zahorsky, *Baby Incubators*, p. 27.

104 published, to his disappointment, locally: Baker, *The Machine in the Nursery*, p. 102. It's not clear whether the book was actually a self-published compilation of Zahorsky's published writings.

105 Rotch, unlike Budin, believed: Zahorsky, *Baby Incubators*, p. 54.

105 "obnoxious effluvia" . . . "the nurses were constantly annoyed": Ibid., p. 17.

105 he found nasal feeding . . . "modified" cow's milk: Ibid., pp. 57, 68.

105 Despite acknowledging the overheating machines: Ibid., pp. 29, 68.

105 "Certain 'specialists'" . . . he claimed the mortality rate . . . "Consequently": Ibid., pp. 15, 14.

106 "The feeling of the medical profession" . . . "effort should be made": Ibid., pp. 12–13.

106 "the catastrophe of hospitalism": Ibid., p. 116.

106 "It was hospitalism that made the mortality": Ibid., p. 29.

106 He concluded that unless a baby's parents were indigent: Ibid., p. 133.

106 Fear of hospitalism: As will be noted in later chapters, doctors began to replace incubators with "warm rooms," the idea being that an open flow of air was preferable. A discussion of doctors' fear of infection, and the promotion of warm rooms, can be found in John Lovett Morse, "The Care and Feeding of Premature Infants," *American Journal of Obstetrics and Diseases of Women and Children* 4 (1905), pp. 589–599, and Jennings C. Letzinberg, "The Care of Premature Infants with Special Reference to the Use of Home-Made Incubators," *Journal of the Minnesota State Medical Association* 28, no. 5 (March 1, 1908), pp. 87–91, both cited in Katie Proctor, "Transferring the Incubator: Fairs and Freak Shows as Agents of Change," unpublished paper, 2004, www.neonatology.org/pdf/proctor.pdf.

Notes

Little Miss Couney Arrives

107 **"to develop into a healthy Miss Couney":** "Invention Saved His Baby," *The Brooklyn Daily Eagle*, February 2, 1907, p. 2.

108 **no one would file a birth certificate for Hildegarde:** Certificate and Record of Birth dated September 7, 1926, stamped 10294, New York City Department of Health. Martin listed his profession as "inventor, scientific instruments." While a very late filing wasn't entirely unheard-of with a home birth, it's a bit unusual—and nineteen years after the fact, you could pretty much say whatever you wanted.

"What Took You So Long?"

109 **Annabelle Maye Couney was the one who had purchased:** Annabelle Maye Couney's will, 1936, file 1668, Kings County Surrogate Court Archive.

111 **"Deponent during the lifetime of Dr. Martin A. Couney":** Letter from Anne J. Boylan filed with Hildegarde Couney's 1956 will, file 4847, Kings County Surrogate Court Archive.

111 **Martin, who'd "invented" the incubators, never held:** Patent records from this time are not digitized. Hard-copy records can be found at the New York Public Library's Science, Industry and Business Library. I spent a day there reviewing every relevant year, looking for Couney, Coney, Cohn—and Schenkein for good measure.

All the Pretty Preemies

112 **"Wipe Hall with Doctor's Body":** The headline appeared in New York's *Evening World*, February 25, 1909, p. 2.

112 **"Dr. Couney: It has come to my knowledge":** Ibid.

113 **A physician named Solomon Fischel:** After his sudden death, *The New York Times* reported that in Europe he had been "an eye specialist." "Dies Ten Hours After Marriage," *The New York Times*, October 20, 1913, p. 20.

113 **Solomon Fischel was wealthy:** At the time of his death in 1913, his net worth was estimated at $100,000 (just shy of 2.5 million in 2017 dollars); ibid.

113 **what was now the Infant Incubator Company:** New York State certificate of incorporation dated May 10, 1905, New York State Department of State, Division of Corporations, book 14, p. 218. The three shareholders are Solomon Fischel, Samuel Schenkein, and Henry Kaufman. Mr. Kaufman does not appear in any subsequent records of the company or the shows.

114 **A child weighing under two pounds:** "Incubators Save Babies Life [sic]," *Chicago Tribune*, June 30, 1905, p. 9.

114 **the daughter of the *Trib*'s own editor:** A. J. Liebling, "Patron of the Preemies," *The New Yorker*, June 3, 1939, p. 23.

114 **the *Tribune* began hosting benefit days:** "Ready for Babies Aid Day," *Chicago Tribune*, July 24, 1907, p. 8; "Riverview Park Aids the Babies," *Chicago Tribune*, August 31, 1908, p. 12.

114 **the 1907 fete:** "White City Astir to Succor Babies," *Chicago Tribune*, July 29, 1907, p. 5.

114 **"to succor poor women":** Joseph Bolivar DeLee, "Chicago Lying-in Hospital and Dispensary," Northwestern Medical School Yearbook, 1903, clipping from the collection of Dr. Lawrence Gartner; the founding of the hospital is also cited in "Chicago Lying-in and Hospital and Dispensary," *The Reform Advocate*, March 1902, p. 77.

114 **DeLee had two Lion-type incubators; by 1902, he had four:** Lawrence M. Gartner and Carol B. Gartner, "The Care of Premature Infants: A Historical Perspective," in *Neonatal Intensive Care: A History of Excellence*, A Symposium Commemorating Child Health Day, NIH Publication No. 92-2786 (Bethesda, MD: National Institutes of Health, 1992), p. 5, http://www.neonatology.org/classics/nic.nih1985.pdf.

114 **He would end up turning . . . Dr. Isaac Abt:** Gerald M. Oppenheimer, "Prematurity as a Public Health Problem: US Policy from the 1920s to the 1960s," *American Journal of Public Health* 86, no. 6 (June 1996), pp. 870–878.

115 **outposts like the Wonderland Amusement Park in Minneapolis and Revere Beach, Massachusetts:** *Wonderland Souvenir Magazine* (Revere Beach, Massachusetts), May 30–September 9, 1906, Wisconsin Historical Society.

115 **Dr. Matthew D. Mann and his colleagues:** Dr. Mann kept numerous newspaper clippings about the ongoing contentiousness of the doctors. There was also finger-pointing among those who felt the initial updates gave the public false hope. Buffalo History Museum Research Library, M82-5, Dr. Matthew D. Mann Scrapbooks.

115 **Austere, with a commanding presence:** Alwin C. Rambar, "Julius Hess, M.D.," in *Historical Review and Recent Advances in Neonatal and Perinatal Medicine*, ed. G. F. Smith, P. N. Smith, and D. Vidyasagar (Chicago: Mead Johnson Nutritional Division, 1983), vol. 2, pp. 161–164.

116 **Upon his return to Chicago:** Ibid.

117 **Yet the Chicago physician never recorded:** Julius Hess archived copious papers but left no record of when this friendship began. I suspect he had to walk a fine line between crediting Couney's influence and maintaining his own reputation.

117 **Morris Fishbein would eventually write:** *Chicago Medical Society Bulletin*, January 26, 1957, cited by L. Joseph Butterfield, "The Incubator Doctor in Denver: A Medical Missing Link," in *The 1970 Denver Westerners Brand Book*, ed. Jackson C. Thode (Denver: Denver Westerners, 1971), p. 358. The obituary has some problems, as Fishbein also says, incorrectly, that Couney was at the Chicago World's Fair in 1893 and that Hess was thirty-two when the White City opened (he would have been twenty-nine).

117 **confusion over when the White City shows ran:** Writing in *The New Yorker* in 1939, A. J. Liebling erroneously said Couney was in the White City twenty-five years earlier, which Couney buff L. Joseph Butterfield later picked up as 1914. Still later, the medical historian and Couney buff Jeffrey P. Baker, in *The Machine in the Nursery: Incubator Technology and the Origins of Newborn Intensive Care* (Baltimore: Johns Hopkins University Press, 1996), p. 104, wrote that while there were conflicting versions, most likely their meeting took place in the White City in 1914. I think the misunderstanding diminished the perceived significance of Couney's influence.

117 **it's reasonable to suspect the meeting came closer to 1905:** In 1951, Hess wrote that his interest in preemies began in 1906, but he did not say what sparked it. Julius H. Hess, "Chicago Plan for Care of Premature Infants," *Journal of the American Medical Association* 146, no. 10 (July 3, 1951), p. 891.

117 **the 1909 competition for best preemie:** "Prize Incubator Baby of the World," *Chicago Daily Tribune*, September 12, 1909, p. G-2. The subhead says that five hundred "mites" were saved by the "physician and his aides." The article itself states that within the

past five years, some five hundred Chicago babies were saved, noting that hospitals had a few machines, but most of the lifesaving work was done in the sideshow. It's possible they included some of those saved in hospitals in the count of five hundred.

117 **Burton Douglas Stevens . . . Little Miss Couney:** Ibid.

Magnetic Tape

119 **Dr. Gartner . . . highly regarded neonatologist:** In addition to his other credentials, Gartner cofounded and has served as president of both the Academy of Breastfeeding Medicine and the North American Society for Pediatric Gastroenterology, Hepatology and Nutrition.

119 **"His name was Cohn":** Lawrence Gartner, conversation with the author, April 24, 2015. All of Dr. Gartner's quotations in this chapter are from that conversation.

120 **multiple legal documents:** Most are cited specifically in other instances in this book. For the 1904 passport application, "United States Passport Applications, 1795–1925," database with images, FamilySearch, https://familysearch.org/ark:/61903/1:1:QVJG -B54R, accessed November 20, 2017.

120 **"He was very altruistic":** George C. Tilyou III, interview with the author, June 27, 2015.

A Dream in Flames

121 **the Great Fredini:** Coney Island Museum. See also https://thegreatfredini.com/2014 /07/31/thompson-dundys-luna-park-3d-printed/.

122 **"At Steeplechase, if the fact" . . . "But should Dreamland":** Edo McCullough, *Good Old Coney Island: A Sentimental Journey into the Past* (1957; New York: Fordham University Press, 2000), pp. 196–197.

122 **For the 1911 season, he'd ditched the all-white theme:** Ibid., pp. 197–198.

122 **George Tilyou, Frederic Thompson, and Samuel Gumpertz:** Ibid., p. 91.

123 **Dreamland was a disaster waiting to happen:** McCullough explains why it was a fire hazard, ibid., p. 197.

123 **the water pressure was weak:** For a detailed description of the water problem, along with the problems of the spreading flames, see ibid., pp. 204–218.

123 **In the morning, it would report:** "Flames Sweep Coney Island," *The New York Times*, May 27, 1911, p. 1; a fourth subhead reads "Incubator Babies Killed."

123 **Miss Graf had been just about:** McCullough, *Good Old Coney Island*, pp. 208–209.

124 **"at least three other infants":** "Flames Sweep Coney Island," p. 1.

124 **"All Well with the Babies":** "All Well with the Babies," *The New York Times*, May 28, 1911, p. 1.

124 **Martin Couney wasn't quoted:** In 1939, he would tell A. J. Liebling a different version of this story, in which he ran with the babies and doubled them with up with preemies on display at Luna Park; this version would be used in his 1950 *New York Times* obituary. But it doesn't agree at all with the reports published at the time of the fire. By the time he made this claim, Solomon Fischel had been dead for nearly thirty years. A. J. Liebling, "Patron of the Preemies," *The New Yorker*, June 3, 1939, p. 22.

125 **"That the infants who were on exhibition" . . . "purely mercenary":** "All Well with the Babies," p. 1.

125 **had attempted, legislatively, to shut them down:** Although the attempt was apparently made—publications from long after the fact, including Jeffrey P. Baker, *The Machine in the Nursery: Incubator Technology and the Origins of Newborn Care* (Baltimore: Johns Hopkins University Press, 1996), refer to it—there is no remaining legislative record of the discussion or vote, nor is it mentioned anywhere in the Society's archived annual reports. The latter reflect an organization devoted to helping abused and neglected children.

125 **had just moved to a new, seven-story building:** Harold Speert, *The Sloane Hospital Chronicle: A History of the Department of Obstetrics and Gynecology of the Columbia-Presbyterian Medical Center* (New York: Presbyterian Hospital, 1988), p. 158.

125 **On admission, kerosene and ether:** Ibid., pp. 169–170.

126 **Sloane Hospital had one hundred cribs:** Ibid., p. 158.

126 **Babies Hospital and similar institutions were rejecting:** The precipitous decline of incubators in the early twentieth century is summed up well in Gerald Oppenheimer, "Prematurity as a Public Health Problem: US Policy from the 1920s to the 1960s," *American Journal of Public Health* 86, no. 6 (June 1996), pp. 870–878; Jeffrey P. Baker, "The Incubator Controversy: Pediatricians and the Origins of Premature Infant Technology in the United States, 1890 to 1910," *Pediatrics* 87, no 5 (May 1991); and in many of the writings of Julius Hess and his nurse Evelyn Lundeen, which are archived at the University of Chicago and cited later in this book. See also the last note, at "Fear of hospitalism," for the chapter "The Crime of the Decade" (p. 247).

126 **the animal keepers freed their charges:** The plight of the animals was widely reported. See McCullough, *Good Old Coney Island*, pp. 212–231; the book gives a heartbreaking blow-by-blow.

128 **Solomon Fischel's Saint Bernard:** "All Well with the Babies," p. 1.

128 **he would go to Manhattan's City Hall:** "Dies Ten Hours After Marriage," *The New York Times*, October 20, 1913, p. 20. The article details the whole grim scene.

128 **"physical force" ... "in a hysterical condition":** Ibid.

The Forgotten Woman

129 **"It is my earnest wish and desire":** Amelie Louise Recht's 1951 will, file 3130, Kings County Surrogate Court Archive.

129 **Her only relations ... Catholic masses:** Ibid.

Building Better Babies

132 **Clark and Watts debuted:** Alisa Klaus, *Every Child a Lion: The Origins of Maternal and Infant Health Policy in the United States and France, 1890–1920* (Ithaca, NY: Cornell University Press, 1993), p. 144.

132 **"advance civilization by leaps and bounds":** "Our Own Page," *Woman's Home Companion*, March 1913, p. 27, as cited ibid.

133 **the magazine would provide gold, silver, and bronze medals:** Klaus, *Every Child a Lion*, p. 144.

133 **Hundreds of pediatricians participated:** Ibid.

133 **Within the first year, forty-five states:** Anna Steese Richardson, "A Year of Better Babies," *Woman's Home Companion*, March 1914, pp. 19–20, as cited ibid., p. 15.

134 "The baby health contest was essentially": Klaus, *Every Child a Lion*, p. 146.
134 "circumference of chest and abdomen; quality of skin, fat, and muscles": Lucia B. Harriman, "Oregon Mothers Conduct Eugenics Department in State Fair," *Child-Welfare Magazine* 7 (1912), p. 84, as cited ibid., p. 148.
134 Even Julius Hess himself served: "Initial Better Babies Contest at State Fair Declared Fine Venture," *Illinois State Register* (Springfield), September 21, 1915, p. 8.
134 "speed the day when we can have scientific elimination": Letter from Mary E. Bates to Julia Lathrop, March 10, 1913 (U.S. Children's Bureau, 4-15-4-3), as cited in Klaus, *Every Child a Lion*, p. 150.

The Day of Couney Finally Arrives

135 "The Day of Couney": July 20, 2015.
136 the German physicians who'd done reconnaissance missions: Leonore Ballowitz, M.D., and Julia Whitefield, M.D., Ph.D., confirmed that it was Lion who showed the babies in Berlin. Dr. Whitefield visited the sole medical school in Leipzig at that time and tried to look up Martin Couney's academic records. "Leipzig told me that Couney was never immatriculated [*sic*]. . . . According to them, they have nearly gapless records (despite two wars)," she wrote to Dr. Paul Toubas, another of the Couney buffs, in a 1997 e-mail. A search in Berlin also yielded no record of matriculation. From Lawrence Gartner's files.
136 "Perhaps Couney 'forgot' he had a predecessor": William Silverman, handwritten note about Felix Marx's letter, from Lawrence Gartner's files.
137 Julius Hess and a New York pediatrician: Letter from Thurman Givan to Lawrence Gartner, December 17, 1970, Lawrence Gartner's personal papers, and another correspondence to and from same, January 18, 1971, Newborn Medicine History Collection, Pediatric History Center, American Academy of Pediatrics. In addition, Givan was looking to see whether Couney took any kickbacks from doctors; he was convinced he didn't.
139 "the first person in the United States to offer specialized care": Press release, April 1970 (exact date unknown), provided by Lawrence Gartner. The plaque, now in the collection of the Atlantic City Historical Museum, has the same wording.
139 "extraordinary progenitor of a new field:" L. Joseph Butterfield, "The Incubator Doctor in Denver: A Medical Missing Link," in *The 1970 Denver Westerners Brand Book*, ed. Jackson C. Thode (Denver: Denver Westerners, 1971), p. 338.
139 "the forerunners of the modern premature nursery": L. Joseph Butterfield, abstract form for "A Photohistory of the Incubator," presentation to be given at 23rd Annual Conference on Neonatal/Perinatal Medicine, American Academy of Pediatrics, District VIII Section on Perinatal Pediatrics, May 22–24, 1998.
139 Thurman Givan, who said they'd been inspired: Letter from Thurman Givan to Lawrence Gartner, January 18, 1971, Newborn Medicine History Collection, Pediatric History Center, American Academy of Pediatrics.
139 "It would be fatuous to attach deep significance": William A. Silverman, "Incubator-Baby Side Shows," *Pediatrics* 64, no. 2 (August 1979), p. 140.
139 Subsequent academic writings: Among others, Jeffrey P. Baker, *The Machine in the Nursery: Incubator Technology and the Origins of Newborn Care* (Baltimore: Johns Hopkins University Press, 1996), reaches a similar conclusion.

140 **On the seven minutes of tape that survived:** Ilsa Ephraim, interview with Lawrence Gartner, 1980 (exact date unknown).

140 **"There was a big exposition in Berlin":** Ilsa Ephraim, interview with Lawrence Gartner, January 4, 1980.

Let's Pretend I Wasn't There

143 **Martin had plenty of time to walk the grounds:** L. Joseph Butterfield, "The Incubator Doctor in Denver: A Medical Missing Link," in *The 1970 Denver Westerners Brand Book*, ed. Jackson C. Thode (Denver: Denver Westerners, 1971), p. 339. A retired electrician who'd worked at Lakeside remembered Martin as short, stocky, and jolly, and that he spent a lot of time walking around the park.

143 **Most of the city's doctors weren't even aware:** Ibid., p. 342.

143 **Meanwhile, at the eugenic section:** Alisa Klaus, *Every Child a Lion: The Origins of Maternal and Infant Health Policy in the United States and France, 1890–1920* (Ithaca, NY: Cornell University Press, 1993), p. 148.

144 **"to understand an interest":** Butterfield, "The Incubator Doctor in Denver," p. 342.

Keep the Incubators, Please

145 **Every conceivable species of minutiae:** Correspondence related to infant incubators, Panama Pacific International Exposition Collection, BANC MSS C-A 190, The Bancroft Library, University of California, Berkeley.

146 **He had also invented his own incubator:** One of Julius Hess's machines was displayed in the American Academy of Pediatrics; the description is based on my viewing. During the Day of Couney, Dr. Lawrence Gartner expressed the opinion that Hess's incubator was inferior to Couney's because you couldn't see the baby.

146 **Julius Hess was offering the ugly-but-functional best:** A chronicle can be found in Julius H. Hess, *Premature and Congenitally Diseased Infants* (Philadelphia: Lea & Febiger, 1922), p. v, in Julius Hays Hess Papers, Crerar Ms 51, Box 2, untitled folder, University of Chicago Library. One instance of the profession's attitude toward incubators can be found in Joseph S. Wall, "The Status of the Child in Obstetric Practice," *Journal of the American Medical Association* 66 (1916), p. 252.

147 **Julius Hess would save his certificate of participation:** Hess Panama-Pacific Exposition Award, 1915, in Julius Hays Hess Papers, Crerar Ms 51, Box 16, Special Collections Research Center, University of Chicago Library.

148 **teammates who called themselves Indians:** Barry Spitz, *Dipsea: The Greatest Race* (San Anselmo, CA: Potrero Meadow, 1993), p. x.

148 **walked the trail two or three times a week:** "Dipsea Originator Is Motor Car Fan," *San Francisco Chronicle*, June 29, 1919, p. 38.

148 **he persisted in calling his little brother "Dr. Coney":** Even his funeral record (date of death, February 6, 1949) lists his brother as "Dr. Martin Coney," presumably from his own documents.

148 **Dundy died and Thompson drank:** John F. Kasson, *Amusing the Million: Coney Island at the Turn of the Century* (New York: Hill and Wang: 1978), p. 111.

148 **Thompson fell ill, and never regained his health:** "Frederic Thompson, Show Builder Dies . . . Made and Lost Fortune," *The New York Times*, June 7, 1919. According to the obituary, he'd been ill with Bright's disease since 1915.

148 **a premature baby named Anna:** Nedra Justice (the premature baby's daughter-in-law), interview with the author, July 14, 2015.

149 **Typhoid Mary:** Her story appears, among many other places, in Harold Speert, *The Sloane Hospital Chronicle: A History of the Department of Obstetrics and Gynecology of the Columbia-Presbyterian Medical Center* (New York: Presbyterian Hospital, 1988), pp. 171–173. The alias Mary Brown is widely cited.

149 **"who has at all times been most kind, loving, and considerate":** Mary Isabella Segner's will, signed in San Francisco on May 22, 1914, filed on September 7, 1916, Tippecanoe County Historical Association and Library Archives, Lafayette, Indiana.

150 **Charles A. Segner was a prominent newspaperman:** An untitled item in the Franklin, Indiana, *Evening Star*, November 15, 1913, p. 3, states that Segner has been named managing editor of the Louisville, Kentucky, *Herald* after working ten years at *The Indianapolis Star*.

150 **the families' later apparent estrangement:** Although Charles is mentioned in one of Maye's obituaries, there is no mention of him in her will. More pointedly, Hildegarde's will says her mother was an only child and her only living relatives are on her father's side of the family, citing his relatives as far away as Haifa, Israel. But Charles Segner and his children were alive and well in Chicago at the time of Hildegarde's death. Even if Maye was not her biological mother, the omission is rather glaring.

150 **First came the memos:** Correspondence related to infant incubators, Panama Pacific International Exposition Collection, BANC MSS C-A 190, The Bancroft Library, University of California, Berkeley.

150 **Just enough cash to secure a down payment:** The mortgage is recorded as $6,500 in the agreement between Sea Gate Development Company, Inc., and Anabel [*sic*] Maye Couney, registered in Kings County, New York, October 26, 1916, Kings County Register of Deeds. I believe the recent inheritance was used as the down payment.

One Very Short Lady

152 **"She was a very short lady":** Nedra Justice, interview with the author, July 14, 2015.

152 **the eugenically perfect winner:** Alisa Klaus, *Every Child a Lion: The Origins of Maternal and Infant Health Policy in the United States and France, 1890–1920* (Ithaca, NY: Cornell University Press, 1993), p. 155.

No-Man's-Land

155 **one would earn the Croix de Guerre:** A. J. Liebling, "Patron of the Preemies," *The New Yorker*, June 3, 1939, p. 20.

155 **That left the littlest citizens in no-man's-land:** The obstetrician J. W. Ballantyne borrowed the term, popularized in World War I, to describe the plight of the preemie. J. W. Ballantyne, "Where Obstetrics and Pædiatrics Meet: Infant Welfare," *International Clinics* 4, 26th series (1916), p. 96.

156 **end up visiting the Coney Island concession every week:** Liebling, "Patron of the Preemies," *The New Yorker*, p. 24.

156 **He liked to cite the names of famous men:** Martin Couney's list is quoted in many sources, including L. Joseph Butterfield, "The Incubator Doctor in Denver: A Medical Missing Link," in *The Denver Westerners Brand Book*, ed. Jackson C. Thode (Denver: Denver Westerners, 1971), p. 343.

156 **"incubators are passé" and "it is a fact that practically all":** Joseph S. Wall, "The Status of the Child in Obstetric Practice," *Journal of the American Medical Association* 66 (1916), p. 252.

157 **Later, he could have added Sir Winston Churchill:** In writing about Martin Couney's show, L. Joseph Butterfield added Churchill to the list of prominent preemies, although I have not found an original source of Couney himself having done so—possibly because he received almost no publicity after 1940.

157 **Before it was over, the horrors of involuntary sterilization:** Edwin Black, *War Against the Weak: Eugenics and America's Campaign to Create a Master Race*, rev. ed. (Washington, DC: Dialog Press, 2012), pp. xv–xvi.

157 **American eugenics would influence:** For a rigorously documented examination, see ibid.; in brief, see p. xvii.

158 **Dr. Harry Haiselden unveiled the third prong:** Martin S. Pernick, *The Black Stork: Eugenics and the Death of "Defective" Babies in American Medicine and Motion Pictures Since 1915* (New York: Oxford University Press, 1996), pp. 4–5.

158 **He eagerly displayed dying babies:** Ibid., p. 5.

158 **Helen Keller:** Ibid., p. 6. In Chicago, Dr. Joseph Bolivar DeLee of Lying-in was among those to oppose him.

158 **The Chicago Medical Society would finally succeed:** Ibid., p. 8.

158 **frightened parents were writing to Dr. Haiselden:** Ibid., p. 5.

158 **The movie was called *The Black Stork*:** Ibid., pp. 5–6; also Black, *War Against the Weak*, p. 257. There were several versions of the movie. As of this writing, at least one is on YouTube: https://www.youtube.com/watch?v=9m6OCT8YmfU.

159 **newspaper advertisement read "Kill Defectives":** Ibid., p. 88.

159 ***Are You Fit to Marry?*:** Pernick, *The Black Stork*, p. 53.

159 **newborns would be coming from Midwood, Zion:** Finding the hospital and institutional records of babies sent to Coney Island proved impossible, as many records no longer exist and others indicate only discharge, without saying where the baby went. This list was compiled from interviews with the babies themselves, now adults; newspaper articles from the time; and written endorsements from physicians in 1937, when Couney applied for the concession at the New York World's Fair.

159 **a Luna Park ride called the Toboggan:** "Incubator Babies Saved from Fire," *New York Tribune*, August 20, 1917, p. 12.

A Charmed Life

160 **"Appleton—Jean Dubinsky":** Death notice, *The New York Times*, January 25, 2015, p. A-17.

161 **She sat with me at her kitchen table:** Ryna Appleton Segal, interview with the author, May 11, 2016.

The Rise and Rise of Julius Hess

164 **"in the United States the care of premature infants":** Julius H. Hess, *Premature and Congenitally Diseased Infants* (Philadelphia: Lea & Febiger, 1922), p. v, in Julius Hays Hess Papers, Crerar Ms 51, Box 2, untitled folder, University of Chicago Library.

164 **"I desire to acknowledge":** Hess, *Premature and Congenitally Diseased Infants*, p. vi.

164 **Julius Hess used a donation:** Julius H. Hess, George J. Mohr, and Phyllis F. Bartelme, *The Physical and Mental Growth of Prematurely Born Children* (Chicago: University of Chicago Press, 1934), p. ix. The initial donor was Arthur Lowenstein. The additional endowments are detailed here.

164 **In 1924, he had a dozen Hess beds:** Evelyn Lundeen, "History of the Hortense Schoen Joseph Premature Station," *The Voice of the Clinic* 2 (Fall 1937), in Julius Hays Hess Papers, Crerar Ms 51, Box 4, Folder 9, Special Collections Research Center, University of Chicago Library.

A Legend Is Born

165 **Inside, character actors also served as lecturers:** The actor-lecturers who explained the exhibits were frequently mentioned in newspaper accounts at the time. For one, see "About New York," *The News-Palladium* (Benton Harbor, Michigan), June 7, 1929, p. 1.

165 **One barker alum, Don Carney, went on:** "Jo Ranson's Radio Dial Log: Uncle Don to Stage Benefit Show Sunday," *The Brooklyn Eagle*, December 12, 1940, p. 22.

165 **Another was said:** William A. Silverman, "Incubator-Baby Side Shows," *Pediatrics* 64, no. 2 (August 1979), p. 136. The diplomat was George Stewart, who became the American consul in Venice.

165 **The most delicious story involves a British youth:** Ibid., p. 136. The Couney buffs held it to be true, but I couldn't find their source.

166 **"Y'see, with the children out of school roaming around":** "Archie Leach by Cary Grant," part 3, *Ladies' Home Journal*, April 1963, pp. 87, 148.

166 **"Cary Grant was a stiltwalker":** George C. Tilyou III, interview with the author, June 27, 2015.

Alone in a Crowd

167 **the Alligator Boy:** This specific freak, along with Lulu the Fat Girl, is mentioned in "'Incubator Man' Saves 2750 Lives!," *The Scranton Republican*, August 6, 1926, p. 6. I do not know the exact year he arrived.

167 **He used no medicine other than whiskey:** Marjorie Dorman, "Coney Incubators Saved 6,000 Babies in 25 Years; Old Idea, Used by Chinese," *The Brooklyn Daily Eagle*, August 4, 1928, p. 3.

167 **Later, he'd claim he would fire any wet nurse:** A. J. Liebling, "Patron of the Preemies," *The New Yorker*, June 3, 1939, p. 24.

168 **The business was owned solely by the "family":** A sworn statement by Louise Recht (treasurer), dated May 28, 1936, within the 1936 probate file of Annabelle Maye

Couney attests that all shares of the Infant Incubator Company passed to the share-holders cited "around 1922." Kings County Surrogate Court Archive.

168 **"I'm not surprised to hear there are rumors"**: Dorman, "Coney Incubators Saved 6,000 Babies in 25 Years," p. 3.

168 **Mrs. Richard Elkins:** "Incubator Baby Is War Orphan No More," *The Parsons Daily Sun* (Parsons, Kansas; dateline New York), September 21, 1916, p. 1.

169 **Occasionally, he said, a couple:** Ilsa and Alfred Ephraim, interview with Lawrence Gartner, 1980 (exact date unknown), from Dr. Gartner's handwritten notes.

169 **if a rich family whose baby he'd saved:** E. Harrison Nickman, in an interview with Lawrence Gartner, May 1, 1970, mentioned wealthy families giving donations; some of the "babies" I interviewed also said their parents gave him a little money.

169 **He'd been filing as a "personal service corporation":** "Baby Incubator Co. Must Pay U.S. Tax," *The Brooklyn Daily Eagle*, June 8, 1926, p. 14.

169 **"You go where I tell you to go":** "Doctor to Bring Charges Against Overzealous Cop," *The Brooklyn Daily Eagle*, July 24, 1926, p. 1; a similar account of the incident appears in "Doctor Denies He Hit Policeman with Auto," *The New York Times*, July 24, 1926.

170 **"hurried out of his cell":** "Doctor to Bring Charges Against Overzealous Cop," p. 1.

170 **For his day in court, Martin took no chances:** "Cops Charges Fail Against Dr. Couney," *The Brooklyn Daily Eagle*, August 3, 1926, p. 1.

170 **Dr. and Mrs. Martin Couney had made a donation:** "Democratic League Observes Birthday," *The Brooklyn Daily Eagle*, December 3, 1928 (the archived fragment shows as M-1, in what appears to be the want-ad section).

170 **Miss Hildegarde Couney . . . she would finish:** Untitled item, *The Brooklyn Daily Eagle*, September 26, 1926, p. 25.

170 **Miss Couney had been awarded:** Untitled society item, *The Brooklyn Daily Eagle*, August 9, 1927, p. 9.

Send the Ambulance

171 **"Things were different":** Carol Bird, "Featherweight Babies a New Medical Problem," *The Lincoln Star* (Nebraska), July 3, 1932, p. 22; see also Isabelle Keating, "Modernity Is Blamed for Premature Baby," *The Brooklyn Daily Eagle*, June 5, 1932, p. 12.

172 **If a mother was broke, he might hire her:** "9 Mothers, 9 Babies Face Brighter World," *The Brooklyn Daily Eagle*, September 16, 1930, p. 15.

172 **Once in a while, a parent sniped:** Keating, "Modernity Is Blamed for Premature Baby," p. 12.

172 **"Such a grateful boy":** "Incubator Baby Not Immune from Cupid's Heartening Shaft; Or Was This Not Romance," *The Brooklyn Daily Eagle*, July 3, 1932, p. 11.

172 **"mannish" and "hefty" and "prickly":** These characterizations emerge in interviews with Moe Goldstein, the "assistant" doctor at the New York World's Fair, and Jerome Champion, the ambulance driver in Atlantic City, and in newspaper articles that describe her as a large woman. By today's standards, she wasn't even close to plus-size.

172 **She weighed 135:** Elizabeth Walker, "Saving the Babies Who Arrive Too Soon," *Santa Ana Register* (California), September 19, 1933, p. 13.

172 **she weighed 160!:** A. J. Liebling, "Patron of the Preemies," *The New Yorker*, June 3, 1939, p. 24.

173 **"They were absolutely fabulous with these babies":** E. Harrison Nickman, interview with Lawrence Gartner, May 1, 1970.

174 **someone would send the ambulance driver:** Jerome Champion, interview with Lawrence Gartner, April 1970.

174 **The news was like a fly in Martin's ointment:** "Stories of 1-Pound Babies False, Says Dr. Couney," *The Brooklyn Daily Eagle*, April 25, 1932, p. 1.

174 **he mailed her mother a Mother's Day card:** "First Round Is Won by Miniature Babies," *The Brooklyn Daily Eagle*, May 9, 1932, p. 17.

175 **"Feed her 2½ ounces of milk seven times a day":** "Smacks Incubating Apparatus for a Healthy Home Run After Being Born Weighing a Dubious 2 Pounds," *The Brooklyn Daily Eagle*, June 26, 1932, p. 2.

175 **"I think I love her as much as her parents":** Ibid.

175 **In Chicago, Julius Hess was forced:** Evelyn Lundeen wrote of the ongoing debate over whether preemies were worth saving. She documented the efforts at Sarah Morris—the largest preemie station in the country—to increase the number of babies the hospital could help, and noted that even in 1937, it was still turning patients away. Evelyn Lundeen, "History of the Hortense Schoen Joseph Premature Station," *The Voice of the Clinic* 2 (Fall 1937), in Julius Hays Hess Papers, Crerar Ms 51, Box 4, Folder 9, Special Collections Research Center, University of Chicago Library.

The Century of Progress

176 **the red giant star Arcturus kindled a brilliant Deco city:** This news was reported all over the country; for one example, see Philip Kinsley, "Star Sets 1933 Fair Ablaze," *Chicago Tribune*, May 28, 1933, p. 1; see also "Four Observatories Will Help Arcturus Open World's Fair," *Chicago Tribune*, May 25, 1933, p. 1.

176 **Chicago's mayor, Anton Cermak, was hit:** Stephan Benzkofer, "Tell Chicago I'll Pull Through," *Chicago Tribune*, February 10, 2013.

177 **"Flagrant above all other examples":** Ludwig Lewisohn, "The Fallacy of Progress," *Harpers Magazine*, June 1933, pp. 104–105.

177 **extra funding through the Infant Aid Society:** Evelyn Lundeen, "History of the Hortense Schoen Joseph Premature Station," *The Voice of the Clinic* 2 (Fall 1937), in Julius Hays Hess Papers, Crerar Ms 51, Box 4, Folder 9, Special Collections Research Center, University of Chicago Library. Lundeen added that after the fair closed, "the nurses were most happy to return to Michael Reese Hospital [the parent hospital of Sarah Morris], where they could care for the babies in a more normal manner." See also "Babies, Babies, and Babies at World's Fair," *Chicago Tribune*, June 5, 1931, p. 20. Mrs. Kellogg Fairbank of Chicago Lying-in was the only woman on the exposition's Executive Committee, and was helping to arrange funding.

177 **a 1928 text on infant feeding:** William A. Silverman, "Incubator-Baby Side Shows," *Pediatrics* 64, no. 2 (August 1979), p. 137.

178 **"Dr. Schulz":** An untitled item that appeared in the Reading, Pennsylvania, *Times*, June 28, 1934, p. 6, notes that while Martin Couney is in Chicago, "Dr. Schulz" is in charge. Isador Schulz, Martin's cousin, was a shareholder.

178 **he requested that a barbed-wire fence go up:** Internal correspondence of the concessions committee, dated June 7, 1934, refers to the request. A Century of Progress records, Special Collections and University Archives, University of Illinois at

Chicago, Box 144. It's not clear whether the fence went up, but the committee seemed inclined to accommodate him.

178 **Their Nazi friends across the sea would be the ones:** For a thorough documentation of the influence of American eugenics on the Holocaust, see Edwin Black, *War Against the Weak: Eugenics and America's Campaign to Create a Master Race*, rev. ed. (Washington, DC: Dialog Press, 2012).

179 **At its entrance was a picture of a stork:** A. J. Liebling, "Masters of the Midway—II," *The New Yorker*, August 19, 1939, p. 25.

179 **Chief Blackhorn adorned Balbo:** "Chief Blackhorn and Italo Balbo, 1933," *The Electronic Encyclopedia of Chicago*, ed. Janice L. Reiff, Ann Durkin Keating, and James R. Grossman (Chicago History Museum/Historical Society, Newberry Library, and Northwestern University), http://www.encyclopedia.chicagohistory.org/pages/11277.html.

179 **the German airship *Graf Zeppelin*:** Besides being written up in all the newspapers, this event was marked by a commemorative U.S. postal stamp. Smithsonian National Postal Museum, Stamps of the 1933 World's Fair, https://postalmuseum.si.edu/collections/object-spotlight/1933-fair.html.

180 **Martin Couney's Spaghetti Sauce for Newlyweds:** Letter from Barbara Fishbein Friedell to Richard F. Snow, 1981 (exact date unknown), Newborn Medicine History Collection, Pediatric History Center, American Academy of Pediatrics.

Not for Public Viewing

181 **A woman ate a hot dog at a party:** Barbara Gerber, interview with the author, July 16, 2015. All quotations in this chapter are from that interview.

All Aboard the Twentieth Century

183 **One of fifteen children:** Accounts of Betty Lou vary, but she herself wrote of providing for her fourteen siblings and helping her parents in "I Am a . . . ," *Jet*, December 25, 1952, pp 24–28. At that time, she wrote, her income was $250 a week. Robert Goforth, digital librarian at Ripley Entertainment Inc., in an October 17, 2017, e-mail to me, wrote that at one point she was making $500 a week. Additional information about Betty Lou, including the fact she paid for her siblings' college education, is found in Marc Hartzman, *American Sideshow: An Encyclopedia of History's Most Wondrous and Strange Performers* (New York: Jeremy P. Tarcher, 2005), p. 230.

183 **people who thought that Hitler wouldn't last long:** For an excellent chronicle of life in Germany at that time, see Heinrich Böll, *What's to Become of the Boy? Or, Something to Do with Books*, trans. Leila Vennewitz (New York: Alfred A. Knopf, 1984).

185 **"You have come here to see in epitome":** *Official Guide Book of the World's Fair of 1934* (Chicago: A Century of Progress International Exposition, 1934), p. 15.

185 **Halfway through July, Chicago inaugurated:** Press release, July 15, 1934, Century of Progress Press Releases July 16–31, Crerar Ms 225, Box v. 2, University of Chicago Library. The ceremony included a big parade.

185 **which the great Pierre Budin did as well:** Jeffrey P. Baker, *The Machine in the Nursery: Incubator Technology and the Origins of Newborn Care* (Baltimore: Johns Hopkins University Press, 1996), p. 52.

185 **Julius Hess was keeping careful track:** Statistical results for 1933: Julius Hays Hess Papers, Crerar Ms 51, Box 3, Folder 11, Special Collections Research Center, University of Chicago Library.

185 **"splendid opportunities":** Herman Bundesen, infant incubator homecoming script for July 25, 1934, Century of Progress International Exposition Scrapbook, Crerar Ms 227, Special Collections Research Center, University of Chicago Library.

185 **"I should like to emphasize the fact that we believe":** Julius Hess, ibid.

186 **"who have come here for the purpose":** Martin Couney, ibid.

186 **One paper boasted that while Canada had the Dionne quintuplets:** "Tiny Infant Attracts Nationwide Interest," *Atlantic City News*, August 17, 1934, p. 1.

187 **At noon on September 12:** The precise details of Hildegarde's journey are detailed in an unidentified newspaper clipping provided by Emanuel Sanfilippo (the baby's brother), July 6, 2015. Mr. Sanfilippo provided a half-dozen such clippings.

187 **heated to 80 degrees:** Unidentified newspaper clipping provided by Emanuel Sanfilippo.

187 **"the flickering spark of life glimmered":** "Hammonton Incubator Baby to Get New Home," Associated Press, dateline Hammonton, New Jersey, September 11, 1934; article provided by Emanuel Sanfilippo.

188 **"We cannot reveal the child's name" . . . "The child is colored":** Press release, September 25, 1934, A Century of Progress records, Special Collections and University Archives, University of Illinois at Chicago, Box 143.

188 **"lots of Negro and Chinese babies":** Paul Harrison, "New York Letter," *The Brownsville Herald* (Texas), August 8, 1933, p. 12. Oddly, Couney himself was in New York when this feature ran. In 1939, the famous columnist Walter Winchell would write that while the number-one attraction at the New York World's Fair was the Perisphere, "the little Negro babies" in Martin Couney's exhibit are "what make the mouth corners curl." Walter Winchell, "Walter Winchell on Broadway," *Daily Mirror* (New York), repr. *Bradford Evening Star* (Pennsylvania), June 3, 1939, p. 7.

188 **Mobs of people:** William Shinnick, "Jam Fair As Closing Nears," *Chicago Daily Tribune*, October 28, 1934, p. 1.

188 **The Century of Progress made a modest profit:** Ibid.; this was widely reported and factored into the decision-making regarding the 1939–1940 New York World's Fair.

189 **Herman Bundesen made his move:** Bundesen's detailed protocol for Chicago, and his showbiz turn, are found in Gerald Oppenheimer, "Prematurity as a Public Health Problem: US Policy from the 1920s to the 1960s," *American Journal of Public Health* 86, no. 6 (June 1996), p. 872. In her papers, Julius Hess's nurse wrote that some of the nurses at Cook County Hospital's new premature station were trained at the Century of Progress. Evelyn Lundeen, "History of the Hortense Schoen Joseph Premature Station," *The Voice of the Clinic* 2 (Fall 1937).

189 **Chicago's citywide initiative was to become:** Oppenheimer, "Prematurity as a Public Health Problem," pp. 872–873.

"My Little Brother"

190 **"My parents never spoke about him":** Letter from Emanuel Sanfilippo to the author, July 6, 2015.

190 **"This hat belongs":** All documentation in this chapter was provided by Emanuel Sanfilippo, July 6, 2015.

Notes

Sorrow in Sea Gate

192 **Isador was dying and wouldn't last through spring:** Isador Schulz's 1936 will (file 5179, Kings County Surrogate Court Archive) indicates that a private nurse had tended to him in his final illness.

192 **Maye's condition was sudden, and urgent:** "Mrs. Martin Couney, Operator of Fair Baby Incubator, Dies," *Chicago Tribune*, February 23, 1936. The obituary states she had been ill for three weeks. Her New York City death certificate (5100) identifies the cause as cerebral arteriosclerosis.

192 **Maye died on the table:** Her death certificate and obituaries indicate this surgery and her death at the Manhattan Neurological Institute.

"Leave As Soon As You Get This"

193 **The letter that came from Uncle Martin:** Ilsa and Alfred Ephraim, interview with Lawrence Gartner, January 1980. The letter itself and the recording of this part of the interview have been lost. Dr. Gartner relayed the information to me on July 20, 2015. Ruth Freudenthal, the Ephraims' daughter, subsequently confirmed that she came here with her parents after her great-uncle sent for them in 1936, and that they left all their furnishings behind, on his instructions.

193 **No flood of Jews:** For a thorough exploration of the difficulty of bringing in Jewish refugees, see Steven Pressman, *50 Children: One Ordinary American Couple's Rescue Mission into the Heart of Nazi Germany* (New York: Harper Perennial, 2015); Edwin Black, *War Against the Weak: Eugenics and America's Campaign to Create a Master Race*, rev. ed. (Washington, DC: Dialog Press, 2012). See also Laurel Leff, *Buried by The Times: The Holocaust and America's Most Important Newspaper* (New York: Cambridge University Press, 2005), pp. 44–45. Leff contends that even *The New York Times* was not entirely sympathetic. In 1939, the *St. Louis*, a ship filled with more than nine hundred Jewish refugees, spent nine days waiting near the American coast before they were infamously turned away. The *Times* reported on the crisis but did not publish an editorial about it until two days after the ship was on its way back to Europe, remaining silent while the refugees' fate was being decided.

194 **"Why do you want to know about my grand-uncle?":** Ruth Freudenthal, telephone conversation with the author, August 12, 2015.

194 **"Whatever she said is true":** Ruth Freudenthal, interview with the author, August 18, 2015. All of Ruth Freudenthal's quotations in this chapter are from that interview.

The Ones Who Got Away

196 **"The doctor said, 'The boys won't make it'":** Norma Johnson, interview with the author, August 20, 2015.

Playing with Matches

197 **Its planners expected this fair to easily exceed:** *The New York Times*, October 28, 1940, p. 1, called it "the biggest, costliest, most ambitious undertaking ever attempted in the history of international expositions."

197 **"If Science, like Art, is to perform":** Einstein's speech in the rain was widely reported. I watched it on Science Planet's Vimeo, https://vimeo.com/28281530.

197 **General Motors' Futurama:** The depiction of the popular exhibits and the overall feeling at the 1939–1940 World's Fair are informed by two books—David Gelernter, *1939: The Lost World of the Fair* (New York: Free Press, 1995), and James Mauro, *Twilight at the World of Tomorrow: Genius, Madness, Murder, and the 1939 World's Fair on the Brink of War* (New York: Ballantine Books, 2010), along with many clippings found in the Patricia D. Klingstein Library at the New-York Historical Society.

198 **the Amusement Zone was the place:** Descriptions of the Amusement Zone are based on my viewing of the World's Fair photo collection in the archives of the Queens Museum, June 4, 2015, courtesy archivist Richard J. Lee.

198 **"bristling with appendages and cast in crepuscular light":** Ingrid Schaffner, *Salvador Dalí's Dream of Venus: The Surrealist Funhouse from the 1939 World's Fair*, photographs by Eric Schaal (New York: Princeton Architectural Press, 2002), p. 10.

198 **envisioned some of the women with hideous fish heads:** Ibid., pp. 105–106. The illustrated book details the entire conflict, including the angry tracts.

199 **the American Medical Association had honored him:** William A. Silverman, "Incubator-Baby Side Shows," *Pediatrics* 64, no. 2 (August 1979), p. 137. Silverman writes that the gift was given in 1937. I could find no further record of it.

199 **Martin had started early, writing in January:** Letter from Martin Couney to Maurice Mermey, Department of Exhibits and Concessions, January 7, 1937, New York World's Fair 1939–1940 records, Manuscripts and Archives Division. The New York Public Library. Astor, Lenox, and Tilden Foundations (hereafter NYPL).

199 **He followed up with eight references:** Report from W. H. Lynn to George P. Smith (Department of Exhibits and Concessions), February 7, 1938, summing up his interview with Dr. Couney, New York World's Fair 1939–1940 records, NYPL.

199 **He sweetened his résumé:** Ibid.

199 **With permission, he dropped the names of Dr. Frederick Freed . . . and Dr. Thurman Givan:** Letter from George P. Smith, Jr., to Director of Exhibits and Concessions, March 3, 1938, New York World's Fair 1939–1940 records, NYPL.

199 **Many years later, Thurman Givan would write:** Letter from Thurman Givan to Lawrence Gartner, January 18, 1971, Newborn Medicine History Collection, Pediatric History Center, American Academy of Pediatrics.

199 **Both doctors asserted their willingness:** Letter from George P. Smith, Jr., to Director of Exhibits and Concessions, March 3, 1938, New York World's Fair 1939–1940 records, NYPL.

199 **the committee member who objected to the exhibit:** Letter from H. A. Flanigan to President, March 10, 1938, and memorandum from W. Earl Andrews to President, March 12, 1938, New York World's Fair 1939–1940 records, NYPL. As it happens, the two-headed dead-embryo showman, Lew Dufour, did get a concession, called Nature's Mistakes; this one featured animals.

199 **he intended to give the building:** Memorandum from Ruth S. Witherspoon to Director of Exhibits and Concessions, May 19, 1937, New York World's Fair 1939–1940 records, NYPL.

200 **At first, he estimated initial expenses at $80,000:** Ibid.

200 **By February of 1938, that had already jumped:** Financial analysis for Infant Incubator project, February 15, 1938, New York World's Fair 1939–1940 records, NYPL.

200 **"He enjoys a very fine reputation":** "Credit and Financial Comments on [Martin Couney's] Application for Concession," January 25, 1938, New York World's Fair 1939–1940 records, NYPL.

200 **Dun & Bradstreet reported:** Ibid.

200 **a rat-infested mess:** Letter from George P. Smith to M. J. Lembo, March 2, 1939, New York World's Fair 1939–1940 records, NYPL.

200 **the extravagant U-shaped structure:** The specifics of the building are found in an undated press release from Ruth R. Meier, Public Relations Council for Skidmore & Owings. New York World's Fair 1939–1940 records, NYPL. The building was also widely described in the press.

200 **six carpenters "on a job that could easily stand twenty men":** Amusement Control Committee memo from A. N. Consier, March 23, 1939, New York World's Fair 1939–1940 records, NYPL.

200 **forced to sell critical stocks:** Report from George Smith to Director of Exhibits and Concessions, April 4, 1938, New York World's Fair 1939–1940 records, NYPL.

200 **bickering about everything from smidgens of inches:** A March 25, 1939, letter from Louis Skidmore, the architect, to Joseph L. Hautman, on the board of design, relays his client's complaint about the reduction of allowable size from three to two and a half inches. New York World's Fair 1939–1940 records, NYPL.

200 **install an electric dishwasher:** Letter from George P. Smith to Director of Exhibits and Concessions, May 20, 1939, New York World's Fair 1939–1940 records, NYPL.

201 **"lay an egg":** "Incubator Man Tells Fair Solons to Lay an Egg," unidentified newspaper clipping, Newborn Medicine History Collection, Pediatric History Center, American Academy of Pediatrics.

201 **"my nurses are strictly prohibited to smoke in the building":** Letter from Martin Couney to Knox Burnett, March 25, 1939, New York World's Fair 1939–1940 records, NYPL.

201 **"Everything I do is strict ethical":** A. J. Liebling, "Patron of the Preemies," *The New Yorker*, June 3, 1939, p. 20.

202 **wasn't "intricate" work and "came from the heart":** John Proctor, "Beginner's Luck," *The Family Circle*, November 24, 1939, p. 9.

202 **"Are these the same babies from Chicago?":** Unidentified newspaper clipping provided to me by Katherine Ashe Meyer, one of Martin Couney's patients.

202 **"How do they live in the gas stoves?":** "Loss of Investment at Fair Increases Dr. Couney's Gloom," *New York World-Telegram*, partial clipping (date and page number missing), Newborn Medicine History Collection, Pediatric History Center, American Academy of Pediatrics. The article also cites "Where did you get the eggs?" and "Are they all from Chicago?"

203 **"I'd rather be helping my father with this work":** Sally MacDougall, "It's Fun to Keep House for Babies at the Fair," unidentified newspaper clipping in the scrapbook of Katherine Ashe Meyer, with the handwritten date of June 16, 1939.

203 **"My Dear Martin, Now that I cannot be with you":** Julius Hess's letter is found on the comprehensive resource Neonatology.org (http://www.neonatology.org/pinups /couney.html). It is identified as having been discovered in the visitors' book for Couney's 1939 exhibit. I have been unable to find the original.

205 **"I'm a baby of yours":** Lucille Horn, interview with the author, April 12, 2017.

205 **"You don't know how much the help of the incubators":** Julia McCarthy, "Sees Her Baby First Time at Fair," clipping, Newborn Medicine History Collection, Pediatric

History Center, American Academy of Pediatrics; title of publication, date, and page number are missing. The speaker is identified as Mrs. Charlotte Preston of Jackson Heights, Queens. I was unable to locate her daughter, Patricia Beverly Preston, who was Martin Couney's patient.

205 **Moe Goldstein was young:** Moe Goldstein, interview with Lawrence and Carol Gartner, April 22, 1970. In this interview, Goldstein related his medical training.

206 **And here was a fascinating job:** Moe Goldstein, speaking to a gathering of doctors at Long Island Jewish Hospital on July 18, 1967, recorded by Lawrence Gartner.

205 **As far as Moe could tell:** Ibid. In his 1970 conversation with the Gartners, Goldstein reiterated a little more strongly, "I don't think he was a licensed M.D. . . . I don't know what, really, what went on," but, he said, "I learned more from them."

206 **he was in awe of Madame:** Moe Goldstein, speaking at Long Island Jewish Hospital, July 18, 1967. Many of the children became his patients.

206 **the gals from the jiggle joint next door:** Ibid.

206 **Martin had put him in charge of keeping records:** The season results are presented in "Incubator Babies at the World's Fair," *The Journal of the American Medical Association* 115 (November 9, 1940), p. 1648.

206 **The tiniest went in Hess beds:** Ibid. For more on the 90 percent survival rate, see the chapter "Who Will Save You Now?"

206 **"Dr. Hess copied a good deal of Dr. Couney's system":** Ibid.

206 **He was certain the boss's daughter had a crush:** Moe Goldstein, interview with Lawrence and Carol Gartner, April 22, 1970.

207 **a team of doctors came from Yale:** Gesell Correspondence, Martin Couney, 1939–40, Box 21, Arnold Gesell Papers, Manuscript Division, Library of Congress, Washington, D.C. Gesell wrote to Couney throughout the fair.

207 **In some of the photos the infants are nude:** Arnold Gesell, in collaboration with Catherine S. Amatruda, *The Embryology of Behavior: The Beginnings of the Human Mind* (New York: Harper & Brothers, 1945). Dr. Martin Couney, Dr. Moe Goldstein, and Madame Louise Recht are acknowledged in the preface, p. x; however, Dr. Gesell chose not to mention that the setting was a sideshow.

208 **He griped about the "sketchily dressed" women:** Letter from George P. Smith to Chairman, Amusement Control Committee, August 9, 1939, New York World's Fair 1939–1940 records, NYPL.

209 **They hit back with a medical complaint:** Letter from H. M. Lammers, Chairman, Amusement Control Committee, to Martin Couney, August 9, 1939, New York World's Fair 1939–1940 records, NYPL.

209 **He couldn't, and wouldn't, reduce personnel or skimp:** Letter from W. S. McHenry to Fred Schulz, Comptroller's Office, July 13, 1939, New York World's Fair 1939–1940 records, NYPL.

Vision and Hindsight

210 **"I would love to talk":** Katherine Ashe Meyer, e-mail to the author, July 31, 2015.

210 **"My mother was skinny as a rail":** Katherine Ashe Meyer, interview with the author, August 3, 2015. All of Katherine Ashe Meyer's quotations in this chapter are from that interview.

Who Will Save You Now?

213 **more than $100,000 in operating expenses:** Report of the Infant Incubator for the Season 1939, notarized statement from Martin Couney, February 5, 1940, New York World's Fair 1939–1940 records, Manuscripts and Archives Division. The New York Public Library. Astor, Lenox, and Tilden Foundations.

213 **Moe was never paid—he was given a watch instead:** Moe Goldstein, interview with Lawrence and Carol Gartner, April 22, 1970.

213 **they discussed what it would cost to move the concession:** Letter from Walter M. Langsdorf to Director of Operations, November 1, 1939, New York World's Fair 1939–1940 records, NYPL.

213 **At the same time, an official wrote to the Smith Incubator Corporation:** Letter from S. M. Smith to H. D. Gibson, Chairman of the Board, November 29, 1939, New York World's Fair 1939–1940 records, NYPL.

213 **He'd mistaken a previous "deferred":** Letter from Edward Rancizl to Co-Director of Amusements, March 29, 1940, New York World's Fair 1939–1940 records, NYPL.

213 **could they please turn the water back on:** Letter from M. A. Couney to Frank D. Shean, March 29, 1940, New York World's Fair 1939–1940 records, NYPL.

214 **"As you perhaps know, Dr. Couney is well into his 80s":** Letter from George P. Smith, Jr., to Vice President in Charge of Finance, March 30, 1940, New York World's Fair 1939–1940 records, NYPL. The Couney buffs also wrote that the city's health commissioner, Dr. Leona Baumgartner, was giving him a hard time, but I have not been able to locate any further record of this. It might have been told to William Silverman during unrecorded conversations. I found only a note from Baumgartner trying to place some of the nurses after the fair closed: Letter, Leona Baumgartner to Dr. Ethel C. Dunham, Director, Division of Research in Child Development, U.S. Department of Labor, in Dr. Lawrence Gartner's collection.

214 **In the end, they agreed on a plan:** Itemized plan stamped by George P. Smith, April 19, 1940, New York World's Fair 1939–1940 records, NYPL.

215 **The previous fall, when Julius was in town:** "Julius Hess Honored at Fair Incubator Exhibit," *New York Herald Tribune*, October 6, 1939, p. 15.

215 **In July, he entertained Morris Fishbein's son:** Thank-you letter from Morris Fishbein to his "dear friend" Martin Couney, July 10, 1940, Morris Fishbein Papers, Box 2, Folder 1, Special Collections Research Center, University of Chicago Library.

215 **proof they had saved more than 90 percent:** "Incubator Babies at the World's Fair," *Journal of the American Medical Association* 115 (November 9, 1940), p. 1648.

215 **a single paragraph about Martin Couney's incubators:** Ibid.

215 **Moe saw Martin crying:** Moe Goldstein, interview with Lawrence and Carol Gartner, April 22, 1970.

215 **Ten of the foreign nations . . . Finland's closed mid-season:** James Mauro, *Twilight at the World of Tomorrow: Genius, Madness, Murder, and the 1939 World's Fair on the Brink of War* (New York: Ballantine Books, 2010), p. xxiv.

215 **The night that Germany invaded France:** Moe Goldstein, interview with Lawrence and Carol Gartner, April 22, 1970.

215 **the city didn't want it:** I can find no record of Couney's having repeated the offer to donate right when the fair ended; by that time, his relations with everyone involved were badly frayed, and he was unable to retire. Dr. Thurman Givan wrote that when

Couney did retire, three years later, he requested Givan's help in making the donation and that New York City (presumably through its health commissioner) rebuffed the offer. Julius Hess gladly accepted the equipment. Letter from Thurman Givan, M.D., to Lawrence Gartner, M.D., January 18, 1971, Newborn Medicine History Collection, Pediatric History Center, American Academy of Pediatrics.

Winter

216 **"just in case"**: Carol Boyce, interview with the author, September 25, 2015.
216 **"He had the ability to put you at ease right away"**: Betty Boyce, interview with Lawrence Gartner, April 30, 1970.
217 **Dr. Frederick Freed, disappointed at being rejected:** Letter from Dr. Frederick Freed to Captain Moe Goldstein, December 30, 1942, courtesy Dr. Lawrence Gartner.
217 **"When they first discovered retrolental fibroplasia"**: Moe Goldstein, interview with Lawrence and Carol Gartner, April 22, 1970.
218 **a gift from Julius Hess or Thurman Givan:** A letter from Thurman Givan, M.D., to Lawrence Gartner, M.D., December 17, 1970, states that he and Julius Hess were sending money. Courtesy Dr. Lawrence Gartner.
218 **Already, the deed to the house:** Records for 3728 Surf Avenue (Section 21, Block 7031, Lot 10) show that the ownership of the house passed to Hildegarde Couney on May 2, 1941. She sold it on July 18, 1950. Kings County Register of Deeds.
218 **"In the last year"**: Ilse Ephraim, interview with Lawrence Gartner, 1980 (exact date unknown).

Epilogue

219 **At 8:40 that morning:** Some reports have the actual takeoff, on September 26, 2015, delayed by about twenty minutes.
219 **Uptown at Morgan Stanley Children's Hospital:** The depiction of care is based on my visit on October 28, 2015, arranged courtesy Dr. Richard Polin.
219 **skilled nursing, hand hygiene . . . Parental bonding:** Dr. Richard Polin, e-mail response to a question from the author, July 7, 2017.
220 **Luna Park Building 2:** According to Jay Singer, a docent at the Coney Island Museum, this was the location of the sideshow for at least part of its run.
220 **This twenty-first-century gathering:** This was held on September 26, 2015.

BIBLIOGRAPHY/SUGGESTED READING

"Baby Incubators at the Pan-American Exposition." *Scientific American* 85, no. 5 (August 3, 1901), p. 68.

Baker, Jeffrey P. "The Incubator Controversy: Pediatricians and the Origins of Premature Infant Technology in the United States, 1890 to 1910." *Pediatrics* 87, no. 5 (May 1991), pp. 654–662.

_____. *The Machine in the Nursery: Incubator Technology and the Origins of Newborn Intensive Care.* Baltimore: Johns Hopkins University Press, 1996.

Ballantyne, J. W. "Where Obstetrics and Pædiatrics Meet: Infant Welfare." *International Clinics* 4, 26th series (1916).

Bartlett, John. "The Warming-Crib." *The Chicago Medical Journal and Examiner* 54 (May 1887), pp. 449–454.

Blacher, Norman. *Sea Gate: A Private Community Within the Confines of New York.* New York: Sea Gate Association, 1955.

Black, Edwin. *War Against the Weak: Eugenics and America's Campaign to Create a Master Race.* Revised edition. Washington, DC: Dialog Press, 2012.

Böll, Heinrich. *What's to Become of the Boy? Or, Something to Do with Books.* Translated by Leila Vennewitz. New York: Alfred A. Knopf, 1984.

Brisbane, Arthur. "The Incubator Baby and Niagara Falls," *Cosmopolitan* 31 (September 1901), pp. 509–516.

Brown, Carrie. *The Hatbox Baby.* Chapel Hill, NC: Algonquin Books, 2000.

Budin, Pierre. *The Nursling.* Translated by William J. Maloney. London: Caxton, 1907.

Burton, Richard D. E. *Blood in the City: Violence and Revelation in Paris, 1789–1945.* Ithaca, NY: Cornell University Press, 2001.

Butterfield, L. Joseph. Abstract form for "A Photohistory of the Incubator,"
     presentation to be given at 23rd Annual Conference on Neonatal/Perinatal
     Medicine, American Academy of Pediatrics, District VIII Section on
     Perinatal Pediatrics, May 22–24, 1998.

_____. "The Incubator Doctor in Denver: A Medical Missing Link." In *The 1970
     Denver Westerners Brand Book*, ed. Jackson C. Thode. Denver: Denver
     Westerners, 1971.

"Chicago Lying-in Dispensary and Hospital." *The Reform Advocate*, March
     1902, p. 77.

Cone, T. E. *History of the Care and Feeding of the Premature Infant*. Boston: Little,
     Brown, 1985.

"The Danger of Making a Public Show of Incubators for Babies." *The Lancet* 1
     (February 5, 1898), pp. 390–391.

Denson, Charles. *Coney Island: Lost and Found*. Berkeley, CA: Ten Speed
     Press, 2004.

Doctorow, E. L. *World's Fair*. New York: Random House, 1986.

Everett, Marshall. *Complete Life of William McKinley and Story of His Assassination:
     An Authentic and Official Memorial Edition* . . . Chicago: C. W. Stanton, 1901.

"Exhibit of Infant Incubators at the Pan-American Exposition." *Pediatrics* 12
     (1901), pp. 414–419.

Gartner, Lawrence M., and Carol B. Gartner. "The Care of Premature Infants:
     Historical Perspective." In *Neonatal Intensive Care: A History of Excellence*.
     A Symposium Commemorating Child Health Day, NIH Publication
     No. 92-2786. Bethesda, MD: National Institutes of Health, 1992.
     http://www.neonatology.org/classics/nic.nih1985.pdf.

Gelernter, David. *1939: The Lost World of the Fair*. New York: Free Press, 1995.

Gesell, Arnold, in collaboration with Catherine S. Armatruda. *The Embryology
     of Behavior: The Beginnings of the Human Mind*. New York: Harper &
     Brothers, 1945.

Grant, Cary. "Archie Leach by Cary Grant," part 3. *Ladies' Home Journal*,
     April 1963.

Hartzman, Marc. *American Sideshow: An Encyclopedia of History's Most Wondrous and
     Strange Performers*. New York: Jeremy P. Tarcher, 2005.

Hayes, James B. *History of the Trans-Mississippi and International Exposition of 1898*.
     St. Louis: Woodward & Tiernan, 1910. http://trans-mississippi.unl.edu/
     texts/view/transmiss.book.haynes.1910.html.

Hess, Julius H. "Chicago Plan for Care of Premature Infants." *The Journal of the
     American Medical Association* 146, no. 10 (July 3, 1951), p. 891.

_____. *Premature and Congenitally Diseased Infants*. Philadelphia: Lea & Febiger, 1922.

Hess, Julius H., George J. Mohr, and Phyllis F. Barteleme. *The Physical and Mental Growth of Prematurely Born Children*. Chicago: University of Chicago Press, 1934.

Howard, Michael. *The Franco-Prussian War*. 2nd edition. London: Granada, 1979.

"Immature Infants in France." *The Lancet* 1 (January 16, 1897), p. 196.

Immerso, Michael. *Coney Island: The People's Playground*. New Brunswick, NJ: Rutgers University Press, 2002.

In re Schenkein et al. (District Court, Western District New York, February 7, 1902). In *The Federal Reporter*, 113, no. 763. St. Paul: West Publishing, 1902.

"Incubator Babies at the World's Fair," *Journal of the American Medical Association* 115 (November 9, 1940), p. 1648.

"Incubators in London." *Pediatrics* 5 (1898), pp. 298–299.

Johns, A. Wesley. *The Man Who Shot McKinley*. South Brunswick, NJ: A. S. Barnes, 1970.

Kamphoefner, Walter D., Wolfgang Helbich, and Ulrike Sommer, eds. *News from the Land of Freedom: German Immigrants Write Home*. Translated by Susan Carter Vogel. Ithaca, NY: Cornell University Press, 1991.

Kasson, John F. *Amusing the Million: Coney Island at the Turn of the Century*. New York: Hill and Wang, 1978.

Klaus, Alisa. *Every Child a Lion: The Origins of Maternal and Infant Health Policy in the United States and France, 1890–1920*. Ithaca, NY: Cornell University Press, 1993.

"Krotoszyn." *The Encyclopedia of Jewish Life Before and During the Holocaust*, vol. 2. Edited by Shmuel Spector and Geoffrey Wigoder. New York: New York University Press, 2001.

Larson, Erik. *The Devil in the White City: Murder, Magic, and Madness at the Fair That Changed America*. New York: Crown, 2003.

Laughlin, Harry H. "The Eugenics Exhibit at Chicago: A Description of the Wall-Panel Survey of Eugenics Exhibited in the Hall of Science, Century of Progress Exposition, Chicago, 1933–34." *The Journal of Heredity* 26, no. 4 (April 1935), pp. 155–162.

Leff, Laurel. *Buried by The Times: The Holocaust and America's Most Important Newspaper*. New York: Cambridge University Press, 2005.

Levi, Vicki Gold, Lee Eisenberg, Rod Kennedy, and Susan Subtle. *Atlantic City: 125 Years of Ocean Madness*. New York: C. N. Potter, 1979.

Lewisohn, Ludwig. "The Fallacy of Progress." *Harpers Magazine*, June 1933.

Liebling, A. J. "Masters of the Midway—II." *The New Yorker*, August 19, 1939.

_____. "Patron of the Preemies." *The New Yorker*, June 3, 1939.

Lundeen, Evelyn. "History of the Hortense Schoen Joseph Premature Station." *The Voice of the Clinic* 2 (Fall 1937).

"Martin Couney's Story Revisited." Letter to the editor. *Pediatrics* 100, no. 1 (July 1997), p. 159.

Mattie, Erik. *World's Fairs.* New York: Princeton Architectural Press, 1998.

Mauro, James. *Twilight at the World of Tomorrow: Genius, Madness, Murder, and the 1939 World's Fair on the Brink of War.* New York: Ballantine Books, 2010.

McCullough, Edo. *Good Old Coney Island: A Sentimental Journey into the Past.* New York: Fordham University Press, 2000. Originally published 1957.

Monasch, Bar Loebel. *Lebenserinnerungen/Memoirs/Pamiętnik.* English translation by Peter Fraenkel. Krotoszyn, Poland: Society of the Friends and Researchers of the Krotoszyn Region, 2004.

Morford, Henry. *Paris and Half-Europe in '78: The Paris Exposition of 1878, Its Side-Shows and Excursions.* New York: Geo. W. Carleton and Morford's Travel Publication Office, 1879.

Official Catalogue and Guide Book to the Pan-American Exhibition, May 1–November 1, 1901. Buffalo: Charles Ahrhart, 1901.

Official Guide Book of the Fair, 1933. Chicago: A Century of Progress, 1933.

Official Guide Book of the World's Fair of 1934. Chicago: A Century of Progress International Exposition, 1934.

"Official Report of the Assassination." *The New York Times,* September 14, 1901.

Oppenheimer, Gerald. "Prematurity as a Public Health Problem: US Policy from the 1920s to the 1960s." *American Journal of Public Health* 86, no. 6 (June 1996), pp. 870–878.

Pernick, Martin S. *The Black Stork: Eugenics and the Death of "Defective" Babies in American Medicine and Motion Pictures Since 1915.* New York: Oxford University Press, 1996.

Pilat, Oliver, and Jo Ranson. *Sodom by the Sea: An Affectionate History of Coney Island.* Garden City, NY: Doubleday, Doran, 1941.

Pressman, Steven. *50 Children: One Ordinary American Couple's Extraordinary Rescue Mission into the Heart of Nazi Germany.* New York: Harper Perennial, 2015.

Proctor, John. "Beginner's Luck." *The Family Circle,* November 24, 1939.

Proctor, Katie. "Transferring the Incubator: Fairs and Freak Shows as Agents of Change." Unpublished paper, 2004, http://www.neonatology.org/pdf/proctor.pdf.

Radcliffe, Walter. *Milestones in Midwifery and the Secret Instrument.* 2nd edition. San Francisco: Norman Publishing, 1989.

Rambar, Alwin C. "Julius Hess, M.D." In *Historical Review and Recent Advances in Neonatal and Perinatal Medicine,* ed. G. F. Smith, P. N. Smith, and

D. Vidyasagar. Chicago: Mead Johnson Nutritional Division, 1983, vol. 2, pp. 161–164.

Schaffert, Timothy. *The Swan Gondola*. New York: Riverhead Books, 2014.

Schaffner, Ingrid. *Salvador Dalí's Dream of Venus: The Surrealist Funhouse from the 1939 World's Fair*. Photographs by Eric Schaal. New York: Princeton Architectural Press, 2002.

Schenkein, Samuel, and Martin Coney. Letter to the editors, *The Lancet* 2, no. 744 (September 18, 1897).

Silverman, William A. "Incubator-Baby Side Shows." *Pediatrics* 64, no. 2 (August 1979), pp. 127–141.

_____. "Postscript to Incubator-Baby Side Shows." *Pediatrics* 66, no. 3 (September 1980), pp. 474–475.

_____. *Retrolental Fibroplasia: A Modern Parable*. New York: Grune & Stratton, 1980.

_____. *Where's the Evidence? Debates in Modern Medicine*. Oxford: Oxford University Press, 1998.

Smith, James Walter. "Baby Incubators." *The Strand Magazine* (London) 12 (July–December 1896), pp. 770–776.

"Some Medical Aspects of the Pan American Exposition: Infant Incubators." *Buffalo Medical Journal* 57, no. 1 (August 1901), p. 56.

Speert, Harold. *The Sloane Hospital Chronicle: A History of the Department of Obstetrics and Gynecology of the Columbia-Presbyterian Medical Center*. New York: Presbyterian Hospital, 1988. Originally published Philadelphia: F. A. Davis, 1963.

Spitz, Barry. *Dipsea: The Greatest Race*. San Anselmo, CA: Potrero Meadow, 1993.

Stuart, Frances H. "De Lion Incubator at Low Maternity Hospital." *Brooklyn Medical Journal* 15 (1901), pp. 346–349.

"The Use of Incubators for Infants." *The Lancet* 1 (May 29, 1897), pp. 1490–1491.

"The Victorian Era Exhibition at Earl's Court." *The Lancet* 2 (July 17, 1897), pp. 161–162.

Voorhees, James D. "The Care of Premature Babies in Incubators." *Archives of Pediatrics* 17 (1900), pp. 331–346.

Wakefield, John A. "A History of the Trans-Mississippi International Exposition." 1903. http://trans-mississippi.unl.edu/texts/view/transmiss.book.wakefield.1903.html.

Wall, Joseph S. "The Status of the Child in Obstetric Practice." *The Journal of the American Medical Association* 66 (1916), pp. 255–256.

Wilson, Nelson W. "Details of President McKinley's Case." *Buffalo Medical Journal* 57, no. 3 (October 1901), p. 207.

Wlodarczyk, Chuck. *Riverview: Gone but Not Forgotten 1904–1967.* Chicago: Riverview Publications, 1977.

Zahorsky, John. *Baby Incubators: A Clinical Study of the Premature Infant, with Especial Reference to Incubator Institutions Conducted for Show Purposes.* St. Louis: Courier of Medicine, 1905.

INDEX

ILLUSTRATION CREDITS

Pages xiii, 8: From *The Official Pictures of a Century of Progress Exposition Chicago 1933* (Chicago: Reuben H. Donnelley Corporation, 1933), p. 95. Image courtesy University of Illinois at Chicago Library, Special Collections

Pages 3, 17, 173: Courtesy Carol Heinisch

Pages 7, 62, 130, 147: Collection of the author (page 147 taken at the American Academy of Pediatrics)

Pages 9, 14, 207, 211: Courtesy Katherine (Ashe) Meyer

Pages 12, 133: From Harry H. Laughlin, "The Eugenics Exhibit at Chicago: A Description of the Wall-Panel Survey of Eugenics Exhibited in the Hall of Science, Century of Progress Exposition, Chicago 1933–34," *The Journal of Heredity* 26, no. 4 (April 1935), pp. 156, 158; reprinted by permission of Oxford University Press

Page 16: From *The Illustrated London News*

Pages 37, 110, 141, 217: Courtesy Dr. Lawrence Gartner

Page 43: Photograph by George Newnes Ltd. From James Walter Smith, "Baby Incubators," *The Strand Magazine* 12 (July–December 1896), p. 770

Pages 49, 64, 67: From *The Pan-American Exposition*, illustrated by C. D. Arnold (Buffalo, 1901)

Page 52: Poster produced by Bockmann Engraving Company, ca. 1932

Page 56: Omaha Public Library

ABOUT THE AUTHOR

Dawn Raffel is a journalist, memoirist, novelist, and short story writer whose work has been widely anthologized. A longtime magazine editor, she helped launch O, The Oprah Magazine and served for many years as executive articles editor. She has also taught creative writing in the MFA program at Columbia University; at Summer Literary Seminars in St. Petersburg, Russia; Montreal; and Vilnius, Lithuania; and at the Center for Fiction in New York. She now works as an independent editor and book reviewer.